Sherry M. Cummings, PhD
Colleen Galambos, DSW
Editors

Diversity and Aging in the Social Environment

Diversity and Aging in the Social Environment has been co-published simultaneously as *Journal of Human Behavior in the Social Environment,* Volume 9, Number 4 2004 and Volume 10, Number 1 2004.

*Pre-publication
REVIEWS,
COMMENTARIES,
EVALUATIONS . . .*

"THIS TIMELY TEXT CAN BE USED IN BOTH HUMAN BEHAVIOR AND THE SOCIAL ENVIRONMENT AND RESEARCH COURSES. . . . Provides the reader with a multisystemic view of diverse older adults, their challenges, and support systems. The text opens with universal theoretical perspectives on aging that offer a background for understanding varied critical life experiences in later adulthood. The remaining chapters discuss various aspects of the biopsychosocial and spiritual dimensions of how people may adapt in old age."

Roberta Greene, PhD, MSW
*Louis and Ann Wolens Centennial Chair
Gerontology and Social Welfare
School of Social Work
University of Texas-Austin*

D1475072

Diversity and Aging in the Social Environment

Diversity and Aging in the Social Environment has been co-published simultaneously as *Journal of Human Behavior in the Social Environment*, Volume 9, Number 4 2004 and Volume 10, Number 1 2004.

The *Journal of Human Behavior in the Social Environment*™ Monographic "Separates"

Below is a list of "separates," which in serials librarianship means a special issue simultaneously published as a special journal issue or double-issue *and* as a "separate" hardbound monograph. (This is a format which we also call a "DocuSerial.")

"Separates" are published because specialized libraries or professionals may wish to purchase a specific thematic issue by itself in a format which can be separately cataloged and shelved, as opposed to purchas - ing the journal on an on-going basis. Faculty members may also more easily consider a "separate" for classroom adoption.

"Separates" are carefully classified separately with the major book jobbers so that the journal tie-in can be noted on new book order slips to avoid duplicate purchasing.

You may wish to visit Haworth's Website at . . .

http://www.HaworthPress.com

. . . to search our online catalog for complete tables of contents of these separates and related publications.

You may also call 1-800-HAWORTH (outside US/Canada: 607-722-5857), or Fax 1-800-895-0582 (out - side US/Canada: 607-771-0012), or e-mail at:

docdelivery@haworthpress.com

Diversity and Aging in the Social Environment, edited by Sherry M. Cummings, PhD, and Colleen Galambos, DSW (Vol. 9, No. 4, 2004, and Vol. 10, No.1, 2004). *Explores the impact of race/ethnicity, gender, sexual orientation, and geographic location on elders' strengths, challenges, needs, and resources.*

How Institutions Are Shaping the Future of Our Children: For Better or for Worse?, edited by Catherine N. Dulmus, PhD, and Karen M. Sowers, PhD (Vol. 9, No. 1/2, 2004). *"A great resource for child welfare professionals working in institutional settings, providing guidance regarding the practices found in one's own agency. The chapter authors are notable experts, and their writing reflects this expe - rience. A highly recommended volume!" (Bruce A. Thayer, PhD, LCSW, Dean & Professor, School of Social Work, Florida State University, Tallahassee)*

Women and Girls in the Social Environment: Behavioral Perspectives, edited by Nancy J. Smyth, PhD, CSW, CASAC (Vol. 7, No. 3/4, 2003). *"At last, a human behavior text in which the unit of analysis is not boys and men, but girls and women. Throughly researched. . . . This collection would make an excellent addition to the standard HBSE course." (Katherine Van Wormer, PhD, MSSW, Professor of Social Work, University of Northern Iowa; Author of Addiction Treatment: A Strengths Perspective)*

Charting the Impacts of University-Child Welfare Collaboration, edited by Katharine Briar-Lawson, PhD, and Joan Levy Zlotnik, PhD, ACSW (Vol. 7, No. 1/2, 2003). *"An excellent comprehensive compila - tion of Title-IVE collaborations between public child welfare agencies and university settings at both BSW and MSW levels . . . " (Rowena Fong, MSW, EdD, Professor of Social Work, The University of Texas at Austin)*

Latino/Hispanic Liaisons and Visions for Human Behavior in the Social Environment, edited by José B. Torres, PhD, MSW, and Felix G. Rivera, PhD (Vol. 5, No. 3/4, 2002). *"An excellent example of scholar - ship by Latinos, for Latinos . . . . Quite useful for graduate social work courses in human behavior or so - cial research." (Carmen Ortiz Hendricks, DSW, Associate Professsor, Hunter College School of Social Work, New York City)*

Violence as Seen Through a Prism of Color, edited by Letha A. (Lee) See, PhD (Vol. 4, No. 2/3, 4, 2001). *"Incisive and important. . . . A comprehensive analysis of the way violence affects people of color. Offers important insights. . . . Should be consulted by academics, students, policymakers, and members of the public." (Dr. James Midgley, Harry and Riva Specht, Professor and Dean, School of Social Welfare, University of California at Berkeley)*

Psychosocial Aspects of the Asian-American Experience: Diversity Within Diversity, edited by Namkee G. Choi, PhD (Vol. 3, No. 3/4, 2000). *Examines the childhood, adolescence, young adult, and aging stages of Asian Americans to help researchers and practitioners offer better services to this ethnic group. Representing Chinese, Japanese, Filipinos, Koreans, Asian Indians, Vietnamese, Hmong,*

Cambodians, and native-born Hawaiians, this helpful book will enable you to offer clients relevant services that are appropriate for your clients' ethnic backgrounds, beliefs, and experiences.

Voices of First Nations People: Human Services Considerations, edited by Hilary N. Weaver, DSW (Vol. 2, No. 1/2, 1999). *"A must read for anyone interested in gaining an insight into the world of Native Americans. . . . I highly recommend it!" (James Knapp, BS, Executive Director, Native American Community Services of Erie and Niagara Counties, Inc., Buffalo, New York)*

***Human Behavior in the Social Environment from an African American Perspective*, edited by Letha A. (Lee) See, PhD (Vol. 1, No. 2/3, 1998). *"A book of scholarly, convincing, and relevant chapters that provide an African-American perspective on human behavior and the social environment . . . offer[s] new insights about the impact of race on psychosocial development in American society." (Alphonso W. Haynes, EdD, Professor, School of Social Work, Grand Valley State University, Grand Rapids, Michigan)*

Diversity and Aging in the Social Environment

Sherry M. Cummings, PhD
Colleen Galambos, DSW
Editors

Diversity and Aging in the Social Environment has been co-published simultaneously as *Journal of Human Behavior in the Social Environment*, Volume 9, Number 4 2004 and Volume 10, Number 1 2004.

The Haworth Social Work Practice Press
An Imprint of The Haworth Press, Inc.

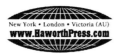

New York • London • Victoria (AU)
www.HaworthPress.com

Published by

The Haworth Social Work Practice Press, 10 Alice Street, Binghamton, NY 13904-1580 USA

The Haworth Social Work Practice Press is an imprint of The Haworth Press, Inc., 10 Alice Street, Binghamton, NY 13904-1580 USA.

Diversity and Aging in the Social Environment has been co-published simultaneously as *Journal of Human Behavior in the Social Environment*, Volume 9, Number 4 2004 and Volume 10, Number 1 2004.

The development, preparation, and publication of this work has been undertaken with great care. However, the publisher, employees, editors, and agents of The Haworth Press and all imprints of The Haworth Press, Inc., including The Haworth Medical Press® and The Pharmaceutical Products Press®, are not responsible for any errors contained herein or for consequences that may ensue from use of materials or information contained in this work. Opinions expressed by the author(s) are not necessarily those of The Haworth Press, Inc.

Cover design by Jennifer M. Gaska.

Library of Congress Cataloging-in-Publication Data

Diversity and aging in the social environment / Sherry M. Cummings and Colleen Galambos, editors.
    p. cm.
        " 'Diversity and aging in the social environment' has been co-published simultaneously as Journal of human behavior in the social environment, Volume 9, Number 4 and Volume 10, Number 1 2004."
        Includes bibliographical references and index.
        ISBN 0-7890-2675-9 (hard cover) – ISBN 0-7890-2676-7 (soft cover)
  1. Older people–United States. 2. Minority older people–United States. 3. Multiculturalism–United States. I. Cummings, Sherry M. II. Galambos, Colleen. III. Journal of human behavior in the social environment.
  HQ1061.D58 2004
  305.26'0973–dc22

2004020725

Indexing, Abstracting & Website/Internet Coverage

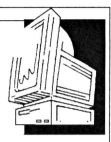

This section provides you with a list of major indexing & abstracting services and other tools for bibliographic access. That is to say, each service began covering this periodical during the year noted in the right column. Most Websites which are listed below have indicated that they will either post, disseminate, compile, archive, cite or alert their own Website users with research-based content from this work. (This list is as current as the copyright date of this publication.)

Abstracting, Website/Indexing Coverage . . . . Year When Coverage Began

- *Business Source Corporate: coverage of nearly 3,350 quality magazines and journals; designed to meet the diverse information needs of corporations; EBSCO Publishing; <http://www.epnet.com/corporate/bsourcecorp.asp>* **2002**

- *Cambridge Scientific Abstracts, Risk Abstracts <http://www.csa.com>* **1998**

- *CareData: The database supporting social care management and practice <http://www.elsc.org.uk/caredata/caredata.htm>* **1998**

- *Child Development Abstracts & Bibliography (in print & online) <http://www.ukans.edu>* **1998**

- *CINAHL (Cumulative Index to Nursing & Allied Health Literature), in print, EBSCO, and SilverPlatter, Data-Star, and PaperChase. (Support materials include Subject Heading List, Database Search Guide, and instructional video) <http://www.cinahl.com>* **1998**

- *EBSCOhost Electronic Journals Service (EJS) <http://ejournals.ebsco.com>* **2004**

(continued)

*Exact start date to come.

Special Bibliographic Notes related to special journal issues
(separates) and indexing/abstracting:

- indexing/abstracting services in this list will also cover material in any "separate" that is co-published simultaneously with Haworth's special thematic journal issue or DocuSerial. Indexing/abstracting usually covers material at the article/chapter level.
- monographic co-editions are intended for either non-subscribers or libraries which intend to purchase a second copy for their circulating collections.
- monographic co-editions are reported to all jobbers/wholesalers/approval plans. The source journal is listed as the "series" to assist the prevention of duplicate purchasing in the same manner utilized for books-in-series.
- to facilitate user/access services all indexing/abstracting services are encouraged to utilize the co-indexing entry note indicated at the bottom of the first page of each article/chapter/contribution.
- this is intended to assist a library user of any reference tool (whether print, electronic, online, or CD-ROM) to locate the monographic version if the library has purchased this version but not a subscription to the source journal.
- individual articles/chapters in any Haworth publication are also available through the Haworth Document Delivery Service (HDDS).

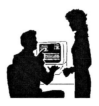

Diversity and Aging in the Social Environment

CONTENTS

ABOUT THE EDITORS

Sherry M. Cummings, PhD, is Associate Professor in the College of Social Work at the University of Tennessee. Her research interests include aging and mental health, caregivers, and gerontological social work. In her research Dr. Cummings examines mental health challenges facing elders in diverse settings including assisted living, community-based, and in-patient. Dr. Cummings has conducted research on depression in community-based and assisted living facility elders, the efficacy of group treatments for depressed elders and for caregivers of persons with early stage Alzheimer's, and on the impact of patient, environmental, resource, and caregiver factors on discharge planning adequacy for dementia patients. Currently, Dr. Cummings is doing research on the service needs of and the efficacy of interventions for elders with severe mental illness, and on the burdens, rewards, and service needs of caregivers of older clients with severe mental illness.

Colleen Galambos, DSW, is Director of the School of Social Work at the University of Missouri-Columbia. She is the Editor-in-Chief of *Health and Social Work* and serves on the National Association of Social Worker's Publications Committee and, is on the editorial board of the *Journal of Social Work Values and Ethics.* Dr. Galambos was a curriculum consultant to the John A. Hartford Faculty Development Institute Project with the Council on Social Work Education, and served as a Project Director for the John A. Hartford Foundation Geriatric Enrichment in Social Work Education Project at the University of Tennessee College of Social Work. She formerly served on the Board of Directors for the National Association of Social Workers and was a member of the Joint Commission on Accreditation of Health Care Organizations Professional and Technical Advisory Committee on Long Term Care. Dr. Galambos has written numerous articles and book chapters in gerontology and has published in such journals as *Social Work, Health and Social Work,* the *Journal of Gerontological Social Work, Race, Gender, and Class, Educational Gerontology,* and the *Journal of Human Behavior in the Social Environment.*

Preface

The United States is an aging nation. The older population (65+) numbered 35.0 million in 2000. Currently, about one in every eight, or 12.4% of the population is 65 years of age or older, and by 2030, over 20% of the population will be in this age group (Administration on Aging, 2002). As the number of elders continues to grow there will be a concomitant increase in the number of elders representing various ethnic and racial groups. In fact, the rise in the number of elders of color will outstrip the growth of the older white population. As a result, the proportion of elders representing persons of color will increase from the 16.4% reported in 2000 to 25.4% in 2030 (Administration on Aging, 2002). While the diversity of the older population is projected to increase, the American Association for Retired Persons (2004) points out that today's elders are already a highly diverse population. Differences in income, health, ethnicity, and social supports affect the quality of life of older adults. A wide disparity exists in terms of income and assets, number of chronic conditions, functional and cognitive impairment, housing arrangements, and access to health care. In addition, the multifaceted experiences that people encounter over a long lifetime serve to differentially shape the quality and context of their later years.

The projected demographic changes of the senior population will raise the demand for social workers who are knowledgeable and have experience working with older adults. In particular, increases in the old-old (85 years and over) population of adults who are at higher risk for psychosocial and functional problems, will amplify the need for support services for this demographic group (Klein, 1996). In order to be more responsive to older adults, social workers and other human service professionals need to enhance their knowledge of both the aging

[Haworth co-indexing entry note]: "Preface." Cummings, Sherry M., and Colleen Galambos. Co-published simultaneously in *Journal of Human Behavior in the Social Environment* (The Haworth Social Work Practice Press, an imprint of The Haworth Press, Inc.) Vol. 9, No. 4, 2004, pp. xv-xxi; Vol. 10, No. 1, 2004, pp. xvii-xxiii; and: *Diversity and Aging in the Social Environment* (eds: Sherry M. Cummings, and Colleen Galambos) The Haworth Social Work Practice Press, an imprint of The Haworth Press, Inc., 2004, pp. xv-xxi. Single or multiple copies of this article are available for a fee from The Haworth Document Delivery Service [1-800-HAWORTH, 9:00 a.m. - 5:00 p.m. (EST). E-mail address: docdelivery@haworthpress.com].

http://www.haworthpress.com/web/JHBSE
xv

population and factors that may affect adjustment in the last developmental stages of a person's life.

If later life development is viewed from a bio-psycho-socio-cultural perspective within an ecological framework, there is recognition that each person has racial, ethnic, and cultural considerations that interact within concentric levels of macro, mezzo, and micro systems (Germain, 1991; Greene & Ephross, 1991). Interactions and transactions within these systems include such entities as society, organizations, community resources, neighborhoods, support networks, kinship groups, family, and friends (Germain, 1991; Greene & Ephross, 1991). Using this framework, our definition of diversity attempts to capture the sociocultural heterogeneity of the older population. Diversity is broadly defined as differences in race, ethnicity, geographical regions, sexual orientation, religion, and health status. It is our belief that all of these factors contribute to strengths and challenges within the life cycle, and present different psychosocial needs and competencies. Recognition of these differences requires social workers to shape interventions and approa- ches that are responsive to diverse client needs. A concerted effort is needed on the part of practitioners to facilitate healthy coping and adaptation with clients to achieve a goodness-of-fit within the environment, rather than passive accommodation that does not factor in client diversity and its impact within environmental systems (Ger- main, 1991; Greene & Ephross, 1991). Social workers are in an excellent position to enhance client transactions within the environment, and assist with the strengthening of client coping capacities to move toward this goodness-of-fit. However, an under- standing of diversity as it impacts the life course is paramount to achieving this practice goal.

Within this volume, diversity and aging is explored through a combination of conceptual, quantitative, and qualitative articles. Each of these articles provides information that will promote an understanding of the complexity of the diverse older population, that is necessary to help shape future practice and research with older adults.

ORGANIZATION OF THESE VOLUMES

The first article by Patricia Kolb provides a context for the examination of diversity issues among older adults by describing and discussing four theoretical perspectives on aging that highlight various aspects of diversity. Stoller and Gibson's perspective emphasizes the differential impact that gender, race/ethnicity, and class have on the shape of the life course. Segments of the older population experience diverse patterns of aging that are rooted in cultural frames, societal structures, and economic realities present throughout one's life course. Friend's theory of successful aging of gay men and lesbian women emphasizes the diverse patterns of aging that may exist among older gays and lesbians due to the varying sociocultural periods in which they were raised, the reactions to homosexuality they have experienced and witnessed, the personal sexual identity they have developed, and their cognitive and emotional responses to heterosexist ideologies. Atchely's theory of continuity and Fisher's theory of multiple stages of older adulthood stress the variety in aging experiences that occurs among older persons in general. Variations in individual personalities, functional capabilities, biological factors, social networks, among other factors, lead to a heterogeneity of aging experiences among older persons. Incorporating such theories into classes examining the life course can serve to heighten students' awareness of the rich diversity that exists among older adults.

In the second article Sandy Butler continues the theme of differential life course experiences among older adults with an in-depth examination of the issues and challenges faced by gay, lesbian, bisexual, and transgender (GLBT) elders and the strengths which they may bring into later life. The various sociocultural periods that have shaped the lives of today's elder GLBT adults are discussed as are factors that have led to the "invisibility" of GLBT older adults in today's society. Butler discusses both the difficulties that many GLBT elders face in accessing services due to widely held myths and misunderstandings about GLBT elders and the challenges encountered by older GLBT families due to legal and policy constraints. The article concludes with a discussion of micro, meso, and macro level practice implications that are particularly relevant for professional and student social workers.

In the third article Charles Emlet focuses on another special population of older adults, those with HIV/AIDs, and examines the great diversity of that exists among older adults infected with and affected by this disease. Emlet examines the impact of gender, race, and sexual orientation on prevalence rates, risk factors, methods of disease contraction, and mortality rates associated with HIV/AIDs among older adults. The psychosocial issues faced by older persons with HIV/AIDs, such as lack of social support, psychological symptomatology, limited finances, the intersection of ageism and HIV phobia, and the lack of existing services for the older HIV/AIDs population, are also discussed. Lastly, Emlet examines the challenges encountered by older HIV-affected caregivers who not only provide physical, emotional and financial support for HIV-infected family members but who also must contend with their own aging and health-related challenges.

The next two articles pick up the theme of caregiver diversity and further this discussion. Nancy Kropf and Stacey Kolomer, in the fourth article, detail the diverse characteristics of custodial grandparents raising grandchildren. The influence of caregiver gender, race, age, and geographic location on caregiving patterns, challenges faced, and supports available are examined. This article also highlights the heterogeneity of the children being cared for by their grandparents and the ways in which varying child characteristics and needs can impact the nature of the caregiving experience. In relationship to this issue, Kropf and Kolomer discuss differences in factors contributing to a child's need for grandparent care as well as variation in the medical conditions, behavioral problems and psychological reactions of these children. This article concludes with an examination of interventions for and public policy initiatives impacting custodial grandparents.

The fifth article by Nancy Giunta, Julian Chow, Andrew Scharlach, and Teresa Dal Santo turns our attention to adult caregivers of elderly, disabled and ill persons. Using a random sample of Californian respondents, the study discussed in this chapter examines differences in caregiver characteristics, service utilization, caregiver strain, and coping mechanisms among racial and ethnic groups. Study results indicate ethnic differences in caregiver health, intensity of care provided, level of financial strain, religious services attendance, former service utilization, and barriers to formal services. Findings suggest that white and African-American caregivers are more likely to use formal caregiver service than are their Asian and Latin-American counterparts. Results also suggest that Latin and African-American caregivers experience a higher number of barriers to service than do whites and Asian-Americans, including cost, language, and service quality.

The following two articles (Part II) give us a more in-depth look at the characteristics of and issues faced by two particular ethnic groups. In the sixth article Morris Saldov and Hisako Kakai focus on Japanese-American elders living in Hawaii and on cultural/religious factors influencing their interactions with healthcare personnel. Traditional cultural values and religious beliefs held by older Japanese-Americans are discussed including dependency on family members, deference to persons in authority, protection of elders from disclosure of serious illness, silent communication, and stoic endurance of illness. Saldov and Kakai report on the findings of a study examining the impact of these cultural values on Japanese-American elders' communication with oncology staff concerning issues related to the signing of informed consent documents. The importance of understanding patients' cultural background and beliefs to prevent negative consequences stemming from unintended conflicts in culture and values is highlighted.

The seventh article, by Margie Rodríguez Le Sage and Aloen Townsend, centers on the relationship between acculturation and depressive symptoms among Mexican-American couples. Le Sage and Townsend, using a national sample consisting of married couples in which both partners self-identify as being Mexican-American, examine the role of acculturation in predicting depressive symptoms. Individual level acculturation is measured through language used for the interview and land of birth, while couple level acculturation is measured through concordance on language preference and nativity. Results indicate significant correlation between spouses' depressive symptomatology suggesting that depression in older Mexican-Americans should be examined within the context of their marriage. Neither individual level nor couple level acculturation, however, were significant predictors of depression among these respondents. The authors conclude with a discussion of the importance and challenge of assessing acculturation when examining depression among older Mexican-American couples.

The last three articles focus on spirituality, an aspect of elders' lives that is receiving increased attention, and examine the differential role that religiosity/spirituality play in the lives of elders based upon race and gender. Holly Nelson-Becker, in the eighth article, poses an intriguing question and asks, Do the life challenges faced and the coping mechanisms (such as religiosity) used vary between Jewish and African-American elders? Nelson-Becker found that while many of the same life challenges were identified by both groups, significant differences in challenges encountered also emerged. In addition, a separate hierarchy of coping mechanisms was found for each group. Religiosity was the most frequent coping mechanism endorsed by African-Americans. Among these elders, religious resources such as reliance on the church community, prayer, and the bible were used more frequently than were social or personal resources. Jewish elders, however, seldom cited the use of religious resources but rather endorsed the use of personal coping mechanisms such as dependence on self, acceptance, and personal strength. Such findings suggest a fundamental difference in the role that religiosity plays in the lives of these elders. These findings also highlight the import of practitioners, and researchers' knowledge of and sensitivity to the varied natural coping mechanisms utilized by different racial and ethnic groups of older adults.

In the ninth article, Roff, Klemmack, Parker, Koenig, Crowther, Baker, and Allman explore both race and gender differences in religiosity in their study "Depression and Religiosity in African American and White Community-Dwelling Adults." The researchers found that females reported higher levels of depression than did males while African-Americans reported fewer depressive symptoms than did their white counterparts. Almost half of the sample were highly religious and results indicate that highly religious persons had significantly lower levels of depression even when controlling for other variables. In the final analysis the predictive value of religiosity overshadowed that of both race and gender. The importance of conducting spiritual assessments when working with older clients dealing with or at risk for depression is discussed.

In the tenth and last article, Yoon and Lee extend the exploration of racial difference in the relationship between religiosity and psychological well-being to the rural elderly. Yoon and Lee discuss both the characteristics of life among the rural elderly and the role of religiosity among diverse elders. In the study, Yoon and Lee found significant racial differences in dimensions of religiosity reported, with Native Americans using more religious/spiritual coping skills than both African-American and white elderly, and African-American elders using religious coping skills more frequently than their white counterparts. African-American and Native American elders also engaged in more religious activities than did white elderly. Contrary to the findings of Roff and colleagues, in Yoon and Lee's study no significant differences in depression scores emerged by race. However, similar to the findings of Roff et al., among the rural subjects studied by Yoon and Lee, dimensions of religiosity also emerged as significant predictors of respondents' subjective well-being. This article highlights the importance of extending research to include elders living in diverse geographic settings.

Taken together, the articles in these two special volumes highlight and address the multidimensional nature of diversity in later life. The articles demonstrate how variations in race, ethnicity, gender, geography, sexual orientation, and life histories may lead to differential values, communication styles, risks, resiliencies, and experiences of later life. It is essential that social workers and other professionals working with older adults and their families be cognizant of the rich diversity that exists within the older population and the impact that issues of diversity may have on their older clients' needs, resources, and perceptions of services offered. In order to effectively meet the needs and promote the well-being of older adults and their families, it is crucial that professionals tailor their work with and develop programs and services for older adults in a manner that acknowledges, honors, and responds to the diverse realities of elders' lives.

Sherry M.Cummings
Colleen Galambos

REFERENCES

Administration on Aging (2002). *A profile of older Americans.* Washington, DC: U.S. Department of Health and Human Services.

American Association of Retired Persons (2004). *A portrait of older minorities.* Available <*http://research.aarp.org/general/portmino.html*>. 2/6/04.

Germain, C. B. (1991). *Human behavior in the social environment.* New York: Columbia University Press.

Greene, R. R., & Ephross, P. H. (1991). *Human behavior theory and social work practice.* New York: Aldine De Gruyter.

Klein, S. M. (Ed.) (1996). *A national agenda for geriatric education: White papers.* Rockville, MD: Health Resources and Services Administration.

PART I

THEORY

Theories of Aging
and Social Work Practice
with Sensitivity to Diversity:
Are There Useful Theories?

Patricia J. Kolb

SUMMARY. Aging experiences are multidimensional, and social workers need to know theoretical perspectives on aging which are useful in understanding the diversity of experiences of individuals in later adulthood. This article describes and discusses four theoretical perspectives on aging which are not usually presented in Human Behavior and

Patricia J. Kolb, MSSA, MA, PhD, ACSW, is Assistant Professor, Fieldwork Coordinator, P.I. and Project Director, Lehman College Social Work Program Hartford/CSWE; Gerorich Curriculum Development Project: Geriatric Enrichment of the Lehman College Baccalaureate Social Work Program, CUNY.

An earlier version of this paper was presented as a workshop session at the Association for Gerontology in Higher Education 27th Annual Meeting and Educational Leadership Conference, February 23, 2001, in San Jose, CA.

[Haworth co-indexing entry note]: "Theories of Aging and Social Work Practice with Sensitivity to Diversity: Are There Useful Theories?" Kolb, Patricia J. Co-published simultaneously in *Journal of Human Behavior in the Social Environment* (The Haworth Social Work Practice Press, an imprint of The Haworth Press, Inc.) Vol. 9, No. 4, 2004, pp. 3-24; and: *Diversity and Aging in the Social Environment* (eds: Sherry M. Cummings, and Colleen Galambos) The Haworth Social Work Practice Press, an imprint of The Haworth Press, Inc., 2004, pp. 3-24. Single or multiple copies of this article are available for a fee from The Haworth Document Delivery Service [1-800-HAWORTH, 9:00 a.m. - 5:00 p.m. (EST). E-mail address: docdelivery@ haworthpress. com].

Digital Object Identifier: 10.1300/J137v09n04_01

the Social Environment textbooks but which contribute to understanding of diversity in later adulthood: Atchley's continuity theory; Fisher's age-independent periods; Stoller and Gibson's perspectives on gender, race and ethnicity, class, and the life course; and Friend's theory of successful aging of gay men and lesbian women. *[Article copies available for a fee from The Haworth Document Delivery Service: 1-800-HAWORTH. E-mail address: <docdelivery@haworthpress.com> Website: <http://www. Haworth Press.com> © 2004 by The Haworth Press, Inc. All rights reserved.]*

KEYWORDS. Gerontological theories, ethnicity, gender, race, sexual orientation, social class

INTRODUCTION

With the increasing proportion of older adults in the population, there is a "demographic imperative" for provision of social work services to a larger and increasingly diverse population of older adults (Council on Social Work Education, 2001). Theoretical perspectives summarized in this article indicate that useful perspectives exist, but textbooks for required Human Behavior and the Social Environment courses often do not include these perspectives. Few theoretical approaches regarding aging may be included, and theories in these textbooks tend to be those which are universalistic, such as activity theory, disengagement theory, and Erikson's psychosocial theory, and often fail to adequately address diversity of experiences in later adulthood.

Universalistic theories propose that experiences of all people in a group are the same, failing to acknowledge the diversity of experiences within a group. As Berger, McBreen, and Rifkin (1996) have indicated, stage theories, or "life cycle" models of individual development, often view human development in terms of "fixed, universal, and sequential stages of human development" (pp. 130-131), and Germain (1994), as quoted in Berger, McBreen, and Rifkin (1996), noted that family development models "do not take into account cultural and historical contexts, variations in sexual orientation, and the influence of poverty and oppression" (p. 131). Consistent with these perspectives, Moody (1988) has suggested that it is impossible to develop an overarching theory of aging because aging is inherently multidimensional. He has proposed that since people are multifaceted biological, psychological, social, and spiritual beings, a single theory of aging is unlikely to include all of the areas relevant to understanding later adulthood. Consistent with this view, social workers need to be familiar with many theories of aging, especially those that explain and validate diversity in the experiences of older adults.

In order to meet this need, this article describes four theoretical perspectives that address diversity of experiences in aging and includes discussion of their implications for social work practice and research: Atchley's continuity theory; Fisher's theory of age-independent periods; Stoller and Gibson's perspectives on gender, race, ethnicity, class, and the life course; and Friend's theory of successful aging of gay men and lesbian women. Discussion of these theoretical perspectives as they relate to diversity of experiences pertaining to ethnicity, gender, race, sexual orientation, and social class in later adulthood is often missing from textbooks for required Human Behavior and the Social Environment courses. Atchley's continuity theory and Stoller and Gibson's life course perspectives are included in some social gerontology textbooks (Atchley, 2000; Stoller & Gibson, 2000), but social work students are unlikely to read these textbooks unless they enroll in a social gerontology course.

Inclusion of content that explains and validates diversity in the experiences of older adults is consistent with purposes identified by the Council on Social Work Education (CSWE, 2003) for Human Behavior and the Social Environment courses. In accordance with CSWE's stated purposes, education about diversity in later adulthood promotes understanding of people from diverse backgrounds and the complex relationships between cultural and personal identity, as well as educating students about interactions between individuals and other systems and ways that systems promote or deter the health and well-being of individuals. Content on perspectives about diversity in later adulthood also supports the CSWE mandate to prepare social workers for practice with knowledge and skills relevant to age, culture, ethnicity, national origin, race, sex, and sexual orientation, as well as the CSWE mandate to integrate content on populations-at-risk and to recognize intergroup and intragroup diversity influencing social work practice and research.

As noted previously, the four theoretical perspectives included in this article have been selected because they approach diversity in aging experiences in ways often missing from Human Behavior and the Social Environment textbooks. I reviewed the following books which are included in Table 1, and the only textbook which included any of the theories was Austrian's, which included all four. Textbooks reviewed are:

TABLE 1. Inclusion of Atchley's Continuity Theory, Fisher's Age-Independent Periods, Friend's Successful Aging, and Stoller and Gibson's Life Course Theory

TEXTBOOKS	THEORY INCLUSION
Ashford, Lecroy, and Lortie (2001)	None of these perspectives
Austrian (2002)	All of these perspectives
Berger, McBreen, and Rifkin (1996)	None of these perspectives
Hutchinson (2003), 2 volumes	None of these perspectives
Longres (2000)	None of these perspectives
Norlin, Chess, Dale, and Smith (2003)	None of these perspectives
Robbins, Chatterjee, and Canda (1998)	None of these perspectives
Schriver (2001)	None of these perspectives
Zastrow and Kirst-Ashman (2001)	None of these perspectives

Ashford, Lecroy, and Lortie (2001), *Human Behavior in the Social Environment: A Multidimensional Perspective*; Austrian (2002), *Developmental Theories Through the Life Cycle*; Berger, McBreen, and Rifkin (1996), *Human Behavior: A Perspective for the Helping Professions*; Hutchison (2003), *Dimensions of Human Behavior: The Changing Life Course* and *Dimensions of Human Behavior: Person and Environment*; Longres (2000), *Human Behavior in the Social Environment*; Norlin, Chess, Dale, and Smith (2003), *Human Behavior and the Social Environment: Social Systems Theory*; Robbins, Chatterjee, and Canda (1998), *Contemporary Human Behavior Theory: A Critical Perspective*; Schriver (2001), *Human Behavior and the Social Environment: Shifting Paradigms in Essential Knowledge for Social Work Practice*; Zastrow and Kirst-Ashman (2001), *Understanding Human Behavior and the Social Environment*.

THEORETICAL PERSPECTIVES

Robert C. Atchley: Continuity Theory

In the Ohio Longitudinal Study of Aging and Adaptation (OLSSA) conducted from 1975 to 1995, deliberate efforts were made by Atchley and his colleagues to learn about diversity of experiences of people in a small Ohio college town as they went through the retirement transition. The study began with over 1,000 respondents and was designed to include all people who were age 50 or over living in the town; 335 respondents were still participating at its conclusion. Longitudinal data was used to identify continuity, stability, and discontinuity in their experiences as they became older.

The information obtained encompassed a broad spectrum. Atchley (1999) and his colleagues learned about beliefs, attitudes, values, goals, motives, emotions, temperament, household composition, marital status, number of children, occupation, employment status, leisure activities, involvement in community organizations, and involvement with family and friends. Background information about race, gender, age, religious affiliation, and education was also obtained, and questions addressed health and disability, retirement, widowhood, and financial resources.

The results demonstrated that there were both positive and negative changes in the lives of study participants in many aspects of development, aging, and adaptation. Atchley (1999) noted that often development was a growth process in spite of modest physical and psychological declines with age, and physical health and psychological outlook improved for some participants as they grew older. A large majority adapted well to the changes they experienced from 1975 to 1995, and lifestyle consequences of social aging were generally minor.

Atchley (1999) developed continuity theory to meet the need for an organizing framework within gerontology. According to this view, continuity exists in adult development and adaptation, as most people continuously learn from their life experiences and intentionally continue to grow and evolve in their chosen directions. Atchley suggested that continuity theory explains why physical, psychological, social well-being, and satisfying relationships and lifestyles are maintained by a large majority of aging adults in spite of living in a youth-oriented and ageist society. In spite of significant changes in health, functioning, and social circumstances, many older adults experience considerable consistency in their thinking, activities, living arrangements, and social relationships.

Continuity theory addresses diversity of experiences in later adulthood in its emphasis that adaptation in aging occurs in unique ways. Atchley (1999) described continuity as the persistence of individuals' general patterns and not as sameness in details of the patterns. Continuity theory proposes that continuity and change usually exist simultaneously for individuals, as changes within individuals and/or their lifestyle tend to be consistent with past experiences. For example, Atchley suggested that an artist who has been drawing for many years and changes to printmaking is demonstrating continuity in commitment to art as an aspect of self and lifestyle. He suggested that it is important to assess the relative balance between continuity and change for people at different times, over time, and during life transitions, and that it is important to assess the extent of the desire for continuity as a motivator in decision-making related to goal-seeking and adaptation to age-related and other life changes.

According to Atchley (1999), two types of patterns indicate continuity: (1) lack of change and (2) only minor changes within general patterns. In contrast, when there are patterns of discontinuity, there are dramatic shifts such as cessation of an activity. He emphasizes that his perspective on discontinuity does not reflect minor fluctuations within past patterns, but significant departures from former patterns.

Continuity theory is also about the development and maintenance of adaptive capacity over time, and construction and use of enduring patterns so that life satisfaction and adaptation to change are enhanced. Continuity theory presents an approach that helps to explain how a majority of persons experience aging positively and as a gentle slope in spite of modestly negative effects of aging on physical and mental functioning, stereotypes about the extent and degree of negative effects of aging, and age discrimination within social institutions.

Atchley did not develop continuity theory as a theory of successful aging or as a deterministic theory predicting specific outcomes. It does not predict that successful adaptation will result from using a continuity strategy but that continuity is the first adaptive strategy of most people. Furthermore, Atchley points out that the results may not be positive, suggesting that even people with low self-esteem, abusive relationships, and poor social adaptation can be resistant to abandoning their internal and external frameworks.

Atchley (1999) suggested that continuity theory is applicable to practice because it helps us understand why individuals have developed as they have and whether or not they have adapted well. Continuity theory "provides a conceptual way of organizing the search for coherence in life stories and of understanding the dynamics that produce basic story lines, but continuity theory has no ideology concerning which stories are 'right' or 'successful' " (p. 7). In order to use continuity theory, information on a person's dimensions including idea patterns, lifestyle, personal goals, and adaptive capacity over time is required.

Atchley's continuity theory relates to diversity in later adulthood in several ways. As a theory based on a longitudinal study lasting 20 years, it highlights the relationship between the experiences of individuals in middle age and later adulthood, identifying many variations in adult patterns among individuals. His research population was a diverse sample intended to include all people age 50 and over in the town. According to Atchley, this sample was selected because there is a tendency to recognize differences, individuality, in younger people, but to forget that differences also exist among older persons. Continuity exists, but many people have the capacity to grow and change throughout life, and personal changes occur in different ways during adult growth and development. Diversity exists in lifestyles, but individuals may want continuity with preferred earlier lifestyles or variations of these as they become older.

James Fisher: Age-Independent Periods of Older Adulthood

Fisher (1993) developed a framework of developmental changes occurring during older adulthood because he believed that no systematic way of identifying and describing periods of retirement with different goals and levels of autonomy had been developed, as well as there not being an approach incorporating the richness and the heterogeneity of older adults' experiences into a systematic framework. It has been noted that Atchley did not develop continuity theory as a theory of successful aging and, similarly, Fisher presented his model as an alternative to models that have the purpose of describing successful aging and which he considered prescriptive rather than descriptive.

Fisher (1993) described older adulthood in five age-independent periods in order to provide a framework for understanding older adult development. He theorized that developmental change occurs during older adulthood in a pattern of stability alternating with two major transitional periods. The periods proposed by Fisher are: (1) continuity with middle age; (2) an early transition; (3) a revised life-style; (4) a later transition; and (5) a final period. He suggested that this framework could be used to identify the needs of older adults in particular periods of development and had the potential to assist in targeting educational and other programs more precisely for subpopulations of older people. Consistent with Atchley's continuity theory, Fisher proposed that there may be continuity in experiences, and these continuing experiences vary for individuals. He also allows for diversity of experiences, suggesting that there are variations in these patterns for different people.

According to Fisher (1993), with the increased number of years and proportion of life lived as an older adult, activities and events have become more diversified and some individuals begin their older adult years with a middle-aged lifestyle. In a study conducted by Fisher, continuity with middle age was described by some people as similar to middle age, but without employment. For these persons, activities included relaxation, sleeping late, travel, activities including golf and gardening, and volunteer work. For a second group, continuity with middle age meant that responsibilities continued to exist. Most of the activities of persons who experienced continuity had been learned earlier in their lives.

For the participants in Fisher's study, the move to the early transition period was most often initiated by the death of one's spouse, onset of poor health, or the need to relocate. Sometimes early transition was the result of accumulated losses related to death of a spouse or caregiving for relatives. Some of the events were experienced involuntarily and others, such as seeking part-time paid employment, volunteer work, or relationships, were the result of personal decisions. Fisher suggested that the events and choices during early transition moved older adulthood in a new direction, that the precipitated process resembled five tasks identified by Clark and Anderson (1967) as necessary in the United States for adaptation in later adulthood and old age: recognition of aging and definition of instrumental limitations, redefinition of physical and social life space, substitution of alternative sources of need satisfaction, reassessment of criteria for evaluation of the self, and reintegration of values and life goals. This transition appeared to be the introduction to older adulthood for the participants in Fisher's study.

Fisher (1993) has described the third period of developmental change as "living out the responses to the events of the early transition and enacting the adaptive choices the participants made" (p. 83). They generally adapted and continued to maintain their independence and control over their lives. Many continued with the same kinds of activities. Some affiliated with other older adults for socialization, and for some, organizational membership was a way to achieve their goals. Life-style changes were highly individualized, and some adapted to changes very positively.

The transition to a fourth period was described by Fisher as resulting primarily from loss of health and mobility and necessitated establishing new goals and activities. Some participants moved from greater independence to dependence voluntarily through actions such as application to a retirement community while they were still active, but most made this transition as a result of disabling events. Diverse changes, including disabilities, illnesses, and accidents, as well as the death of a spouse, a relative's relocation, or the loss of a caregiver, precipitated the loss of independent living.

This was followed by a stable period which included revised goals and activities implemented within a context of limited mobility. Reflecting diverse responses, some of the participants enjoyed positive new activities and growth in settings including nursing homes, but resignation and loneliness were also experienced.

The participants generally described their movement as sequential through the periods, although there were exceptions when a spouse had died before a participant completed all periods or a person experienced a disabling illness before or during the first period and went directly into the last transition period. Experiences of recycling or circling back to earlier stages occurred primarily among persons who remarried. For people who described experiences that followed Fisher's framework sequentially, the periods, beginning with retirement and ending with death, differed in length. He also noted that for women who had experienced little or no employment outside of their home, retirement was an elusive concept.

According to Fisher, if developmental differences in older adults are identified, service providers can develop programs that address the needs of subpopulations. As an educator, he also suggested that this knowledge can provide a foundation for development of education programs to assist older adults to anticipate, cope, and respond to the changes experienced in the stages and transitions.

This theory applies to diverse groups of older adults because it acknowledges variations in the sequence of developmental periods that include skipped developmental periods, recycling and circling back, variations in length of developmental periods, and retirement as an elusive concept for some women who have never worked outside of their home. Fisher attributes variations in events and timing to several factors, including illness or death, which are outside of the control of the individual. However, older adults exercise adaptive choices, and in the third period of developmental change his participants' adaptive choices were lived-out responses to the early transition. When loss of independence was experienced in the fourth period, this change resulted from diverse experiences and was experienced in different ways. Even when participants engaged in activities within a context of limited mobility, emotional and social responses varied within the group. Atchley's continuity theory and Fisher's theory of age-independent periods of older adulthood share an emphasis on diversity of responses to age-related changes with regard to both the nature and timing of changes and adaptation. The life-style changes experienced by people in each of their studies were highly individualized.

Eleanor Palo Stoller and Rose Campbell Gibson: Gender, Race and Ethnicity, Class, and the Life Course

Stoller and Gibson (2000a) have introduced the life course perspective as a framework that provides an inclusive approach to the study of aging. Their approach to this perspective has four main premises: (1) personal attributes, particular life events, and adaptation to events affect the process of aging; (2) opportunity structures are shaped by socio-historical times and differ for individuals based on personal characteristics, such as subordinate social status; (3) the experience of aging is shaped by birth in a particular time period, or cohort membership, and individuals' aging experiences within cohorts vary depending on one's position in hierarchies of class, ethnicity, gender, and race in which there are inequalities; and (4) disadvantaged and privileged members of the same cohort are affected differently by the socio-historical period shaping their experiences.

According to Stoller and Gibson (1997), the life course perspective introduces the elements of personal biography, sociocultural factors, and sociocultural times that have been neglected by earlier theories of aging, and inclusion of these elements provides a broader approach to understanding the aging process. They suggest that when we consider differences within cohorts based on characteristics like race and gender, this helps us to understand inequalities experienced by subgroups within a cohort, including experiences in the lives of African Americans prior to the Civil Rights movement, experiences which blocked their opportunities and required development of adaptive resources that affect members of this group today as older adults.

Theoretical perspectives proposed by Stoller and Gibson are important in understanding diversity of aging experiences related to gender, race and ethnicity, and social class. Stoller and Gibson (2000b) have proposed that gender, race, ethnicity, and social class are factors that structure "different worlds in aging" because there are discernible patterns in the experiences of different segments of the older population which reflect social structural arrangements and cultural blueprints within society. They emphasize that although gender, race or ethnicity, and social class are often perceived to be attributes of individuals, these characteristics are social constructs which are classifications based on social values. They have explored these constructs from the perspective of sociologist Beth Hess's (1990) conceptualization of gender, race, and class "both as labels attached to individuals and as properties of hierarchical social structures within which people form identities and through which they realize their life chances" (Stoller & Gibson, 2000b, p. 4). They also "investigate the ways in which people's positions along these multiple hierarchies generate diverse views of social reality," suggesting that this "involves listening to descriptions of aging and old age from multiple perspectives, of giving voice to people whose perspectives have been overlooked" (2000b, p. 4).

Stoller and Gibson (2000b) have written that focusing upon hierarchies based on gender, race or ethnicity, and social class enables us to recognize elements of discrimination that have influenced the lives of older adults. For example, legally segregated school systems and discriminatory hiring practices have limited the opportunities for today's African American older adults to accumulate financial assets during their younger years. They note that a lifetime of poverty results in poor health in later life and that multiple jeopardy, i.e., occupying several disadvantaged positions simultaneously, increases the risk of negative outcomes when people become old.

Furthermore, systems of privilege are created through these same hierarchies, providing unearned advantages to persons on the basis of being White, being male, and belonging to the middle or upper class, although the emphasis on disadvantage sometimes masks this reality (Stoller & Gibson, 2000b). These privileges are unearned because they are determined by ascribed rather than achieved status. Stoller and Gibson (2000b) explain privilege and disadvantage, stating that identifying privilege and disadvantage can be complicated since people can experience disadvantage along one dimension but privilege along others. They state that since there are intersections along multiple hierarchies, it is incorrect to assume that all men are more privileged than all women or that all Whites experience greater advantage than all people of color. According to Stoller and Gibson, diversity in the amount of accumulated resources, relationships, meanings attached to aging, and definitions of social reality exists for older adults because of lifetimes of experiences within multiple hierarchies.

Stoller and Gibson (2000b) emphasize strengths as well as deficits, pointing out that the multiple jeopardy approach to studying inequality in old age emphasizes negative outcomes of living in disadvantaged positions, but it is also important to learn how older persons experiencing multiple jeopardy also create meaning in their lives despite barriers resulting from these hierarchies. It should be kept in mind, however, that there are clear implications for the health and mental health status of aging minority women which are related to marked disparities in income, including higher morbidity rates for diabetes, hypertension, and kidney disease (Padgett, 1999).

The theoretical perspectives of Stoller and Gibson described in this section are relevant to diverse groups of elders because they address "different worlds in aging," divergent realities in the lives of older adults related to gender, race, ethnicity, and social class. Stoller and Gibson identify these as social constructs and describe the systems of disadvantage and privilege created by ascribed status conferred within these hierarchies. Lifetimes of experiences within multiple hierarchies have resulted in diversity of experiences in later adulthood, and experiences are all the more diverse because an individual can experience disadvantage along one dimension and privileges along other dimensions. They note that while disadvantages result from experiencing multiple jeopardy, persons experiencing multiple jeopardy create meaning in their lives despite the associated barriers. Many older Americans experience adversities related to classism, racism, and sexism in different degrees and forms, and vary in their development of coping skills to respond to these socially constructed conditions imposed on their lives.

Richard Friend: Successful Aging of Older Lesbian Women and Gay Men

Stoller and Gibson have proposed that gender, race, ethnicity, and social class are factors that structure "different worlds in aging," and this is also true of sexual orientation. This aspect of identity is also a concept which is a social construct based on social values. Friend's theory of successful aging addresses the need to develop theoretical perspectives regarding the experiences of older lesbian women and gay men, and this perspective is consistent with Stoller and Gibson's emphasis on the influence of socially constructed identities on diversity of aging experiences. Friend (1980, 1991) and other authors (Francher & Henkin, 1973; Kimmel, 1977) have suggested that because of the experience of managing what it means to be lesbian or gay in a heterosexist world, many lesbian women and gay men develop skills for managing their lives which also facilitate their adjustment to the aging process, and Friend developed his theory of successful aging to describe these processes.

Friend (1991) suggested that common unifying elements for lesbian women and gay men are that today's older lesbian and gay people developed some kind of homosexual identity and grew up in a particular socio-historical period. He adds that research findings disagree with the common negative stereotypes of older gay men as lonely, depressed, oversexed, and lacking support from family and friends (Kelly, 1977), and stereotypes of older lesbian women as unattractive, unemotional, and lonely (Berger, 1982a).

Friend (1991) indicates that many researchers (Kelly, 1977; Berger, 1982a, 1982b; Friend, 1980; Kimmel, 1978; Weinberg, 1970) have studied older gay men who have been accepting of themselves, well-adjusted psychologically, and adapting well to aging. He also notes that research findings in several studies (Almvig, 1982; Martin & Lyon, 1979; Raphael & Robinson, 1980) have found that over half of the older lesbian women in their studies were happy and well-adjusted. Likewise, Kehoe (1988) found that most of the women in her study of lesbians over the age of 60 sustained relatively high morale and life satisfaction.

Friend (1991) points out that there is diversity among gay men and lesbian women in their responses to the social construction of homosexuality as a negative identity, suggesting that people may internalize negative messages about homosexuality or reconstruct its meaning positively. In presenting his theory of successful aging, Friend proposed that when people develop a positive lesbian or gay identity, they acquire certain skills, feelings and attitudes that are resources which facilitate adjustment to aging. Applying social construction theory, he developed a model to describe the diverse ways in which sexual identity is formed by older lesbian women and gay men. According to Friend (1991), a theory of what it means to successfully grow old can be developed by closely examining "the relationship between the social construction of lesbian and gay identities and the individual psychology of older gay and lesbian people who have worked to make their lives meaningful within the context of a particular socio-historical period of time" (p. 100).

Friend (1991) suggests that the process of developing one's identity as a lesbian or gay person reflects the relationship between individual psychology and social construction, as each lesbian woman and gay man creates individual meaning out of messages about homosexuality within the context of social norms. According to Friend, when heterosexist discourse constructed homosexual identity as sickness around 1900 in the United States, internalized homophobia and resistance were two of the responses among lesbian women and gay men. He argues that older lesbian women and gay men growing up close to this socio-historical period have experienced cognitive/behavioral responses to heterosexism along a continuum ranging from resistance to internalized homophobia, and that there is also a continuum of related emotional responses. His model proposes that these responses occur along a cognitive/behavioral continuum ranging from internalization of pervasive heterosexist ideologies imputing sickness and/or other negative attributes, to a response at the other end of the continuum which involves reconstruction of what it means to be lesbian or gay into something positive and affirmative through challenging or questioning the validity of negative messages. There are also corresponding affective responses along this continuum. Friend suggests that if a person's evaluation of homosexuality is negative, the corresponding emotional response will be internalized homophobia which may result in self-hatred, low self-esteem, and minimal or conditional self-acceptance. He states that at the other end of the continuum, a positive gay or lesbian identity, related affective responses include feelings of increased self-acceptance, high self-esteem, personal empowerment, and self-affirmation.

According to Friend (1991), for contemporary gay and lesbian older adults, there is a shared socio-historical context of living a major part of their lives in historical periods in which there have been at least three different groups of older lesbians and gay adults characterized by differing cognitive/behavioral and emotional responses to their experiences. He proposed that their responses represent three styles of identity formation within the same cohort, and more styles are possible on these continua. The three groups identified by Friend (1991) are: (1) "Stereotypic Older Lesbian and Gay People" whose cognitive/behavioral responses to heterosexism reflect extreme internalized homophobia and who are lonely, depressed, and alienated; (2) "Affirmative Older Lesbian and Gay People" whose response to heterosexism has been to reconstruct a positive and affirmative sense of self and who are psychologically well-adjusted, vibrant, and adapting well to the aging process; and (3) persons who are "Passing Older Lesbian and Gay People" who as people in mid-range of the continua believe that heterosexuality is inherently better but marginally accept some aspects of homosexuality, and who are strongly invested in passing as persons who are not gay or lesbian, or not stereotypically lesbian or gay. Friend also suggested that other styles of identity formation are possible.

According to Friend, successful aging for gay men and lesbian women is a result of reconstruction of homosexuality as a positive attribute within the contexts of individual psychology. He suggests that this occurs through development of crisis competence, flexibility in gender role, and reconstruction of personal meanings of homosexuality and aging; social and interpersonal dimensions which include planning for one's own future security, redefinition of family, reinforcing family supports with those of friends and community; and the development of legal and political advocacy skills to directly manage heterosexism and ageism.

Consistent with Stoller and Gibson's perspectives described in the previous section, Friend's theoretical perspective of differences in the aging experiences of subgroups of gay men and lesbian women reflects the idea of "different worlds in aging" influenced by earlier life experiences lived within the context of a particular socio-historical period. He has used social construction theory to develop a model regarding diverse ways that identity regarding sexual orientation is formed. The cognitive/behavioral and affective responses that he describes reflect differences in experiences of lesbian women and gay men compared to heterosexual men and women in the United States, and Friend goes beyond this to propose a continuum of differences between subgroups of lesbian women and gay men that he believes influences responses to aging. He identifies diverse responses among lesbian women and gay men to the socially constructed view of homosexuality as a negative identity and suggests that there are variations in adjustment to aging that are related to whether a person has developed a positive or more negative lesbian or gay identity.

Summary of Key Components of the Four Perspectives

Key components of the theoretical perspectives described in this article are summarized in Table 2.

CONCLUSIONS AND IMPLICATIONS

There are theories of aging that are useful in social work practice with sensitivity to diversity. Atchley's continuity theory; Fisher's theory of age-independent periods; Stoller and Gibson's perspectives on gender, race and ethnicity, class, and the life course; and Friend's theory of successful aging of gay men and lesbian women are theoretical perspectives addressing diversity more successfully than universalistic theories of aging.

Atchley's research findings and his conceptualization of continuity theory have many implications for social work practice and research. Relevant to practice, continuity theory highlights the importance of assessing the relative balance of continuity and change in an individual and the reality that the desire for continuity can be a motivator in goal-seeking and adaptation. Atchley also reminds us that maintaining a

TABLE 2. Major Concepts in Four Theoretical Perspectives

Atchley's Continuity Theory

- There are variations in the retirement experiences of individuals over time.
- People experience both stability and discontinuity as they become older.
- There can be declines and improvements in the physical and psychological functioning of individuals as they become older.
- Adaptation to aging occurs in unique ways for individuals.
- Many people maintain their adaptive capacity over time and use enduring patterns to enhance their life satisfaction and adaptation as they become older.
- Some people, but not all, maintain consistency over time in their thinking patterns, activity profiles, living arrangements, and social relations, but this does not apply to all people as they become older.

Fisher's Theory of Multiple Stages of Older Adulthood

- Aging experiences are diverse and unpredictable due to social and biological factors.
- As adults age, they generally experience specific stable periods alternating with transitional periods.
- People have different experiences within five age-independent periods, and these periods occur at different ages for different people.
- There are variations in the sequence and length of the periods.
- Various voluntary and involuntary life events precipitate movement to the next stage.
- Retirement has been an elusive concept for some women who have never engaged in paid employment.

Stoller and Gibson's Life Course Perspective

- Gender, race and ethnicity, and social class are social constructs which are classifications based on social values.
- Gender, race and ethnicity, and social class are factors that structure "different worlds in aging."
- There are discernible and diverse patterns in the experiences of different segments of the older population that reflect social structural arrangements and cultural blueprints in society.
- This view of the life course introduces the elements of personal biography, sociocultural factors, and sociocultural times that were neglected in many of the earlier theories of aging.

Friend's Theory of Successful Aging of Older Gay Men and Lesbian Women

- The process of developing one's identity as a lesbian or gay person reflects the relationship between individual psychology and social construction as individuals go through the process of creating meaning from messages about homosexuality within the context of social norms.
- Common unifying elements for today's lesbian women and gay men are that they developed some kind of homosexual identity and grew up in a particular socio-historical period.
- For some people, the experience of managing what it means to be lesbian or gay in a heterosexist world contributes to the development of skills which facilitate adjustment to the aging process.
- Responses of older lesbian women and gay men to heterosexism vary along a continuum of cognitive/behavioral and related emotional responses ranging from internalization of pervasive heterosexist ideologies to reconstruction of what it means to be lesbian or gay into a positive and affirmative response.

relationship with longstanding activities can be important in maintaining older adults' self-esteem. Continuity theory also implies support for life review and reminiscence as positive approaches for older adults to identify the strengths, psychological and social resources, and interests developed throughout life that may be useful in later adulthood.

Consistent with the strengths perspective, Atchley's research documented that adaptive capacity is maintained over time and that many people use enduring patterns to enhance life satisfaction and adaptation to change. Social workers need to recognize the importance of these patterns, help people to identify their own patterns that are strengths and resources in aging, work with clients to have the necessary resources to support continuation of longstanding activities, and yet acknowledge and support the capacity of many people for growth and change throughout life. For example, a nursing home social worker needs to recognize that some residents have longstanding patterns of involvement and preference for a broad range of activities involving interpersonal contact, while other residents have a preference and patterns of more solitary activities that may include reading and other tasks that have been carried out in their home. Social workers should inform residents of nursing homes and older adults in other settings about the range of group and individual activities available, as well as opportunities to initiate participation, but respect individuals' longstanding patterns, potential need for continuity, and right to self-determination in choices regarding how they spend their time. Social workers can also question institutional policies and practices in nursing homes and other practice settings that impede opportunities for continuity for older adults who prefer activities providing continuity and try to bring about changes in these policies and practices.

Atchley's study has many implications for research on related topics. These include: (1) studies of social workers' perceptions of whether or not their older clients desire continuity and/or change in their lives; (2) characteristics of clients preferring continuity or change or modified continuity; (3) social workers' attitudes about the desire of their clients for complete continuity, changes within continuing patterns, or desire for major changes from long-term patterns; (4) social workers' expectations about continuity or change in the lives of older adults; and (5) social work practice approaches that support and/or impede continuity or change in the lives of older adults. Studies can also be conducted pertaining to access to formal services and informal support for adults desiring continuity and/or change in their lives, considering variables including size and socioeconomic characteristics of communities, and individual attributes including age, ethnicity, gender, immigration status, physical and mental health, race, sexual orientation, socioeconomic status, and spirituality.

Consistent with continuity theory, Fisher's theory of multiple stages of older adulthood reflects the perspective that aging experiences are diverse and unpredictable due to social and biological factors, and that assessments and interventions should include differentiation of older adults within cohorts. His framework supports program development by identifying developmental differences in older adults.

Implications of this theory for social work practice include the importance of understanding the transitional periods from middle to later adulthood and the importance of social work practice in work with clients experiencing difficult transitions and adjustments to changes. Fisher suggested that the framework can be used to identify needs during particular periods of development and to develop educational programs for subpopulations of older adults, suggesting that programmatic responses can be developed to assist older adults to anticipate, cope, and respond to the changes experienced in the stages and transitions. Understanding the framework can be useful in developing interventions with individuals and groups experiencing difficult, sometimes involuntary, transitions and can support counseling efforts and create linkages with other resources.

Fisher's theoretical perspective implies that it is important for social work researchers to identify needs and impediments to meeting these that are experienced by individuals during the periods from middle age to old age. Research could also yield useful information about the supports needed, available, and lacking in informal and formal systems, providing assistance as people experience changes in different periods. Finally, studies similar to Fisher's are needed that will focus on experiences in developmental periods from middle to later adulthood in groups that differ in terms of ethnicity, gender, immigration status, race, sexual orientation, and socioeconomic status. Issues that need to be addressed include the questions of whether there tend to be variations in developmental stages within different groups and variations in factors precipitating transitions in different groups, as well as differences among individuals within groups.

Theoretical perspectives of Stoller and Gibson and Friend support the view that gender, race and ethnicity, sexual orientation, and social class are factors that structure "different worlds in aging." Their approaches clarify the need for practitioners to understand older adults within the context of the diverse environments in which they have lived their lives. Inclusion of content reflecting this is essential in Human Behavior and the Social Environment courses.

Stoller and Gibson's perspectives regarding socially constructed systems of oppression and privilege and the life course introduce insights about prejudice, discrimination, and privilege that are important in social work practice from a biopsychosocial perspective with older adults with extremely divergent life experiences. As noted previously, Stoller and Gibson remind us that there are multiple hierarchies, and experiences along these contribute to diversity in resources, relationships, meanings attached to aging, and social realities. Their perspectives are a reminder to social workers that issues of privilege and disadvantage are complicated because an individual can be privileged along one dimension and disadvantaged along others. The theoretical perspectives of Friend and Stoller and Gibson can foster development of nonjudgmental attitudes and professional objectivity, as well as understanding and commitment to social justice, because of increased comprehension of the effects, both negative and positive, of lifelong experiences with prejudice, discrimination, and privilege. This knowledge can contribute to social work activism and initiatives to deconstruct systems of oppression.

Additionally, Stoller and Gibson's theoretical perspectives support the strengths perspective when they point out that persons experiencing prejudice and discrimination may create meaning in their lives despite disadvantages. Stoller and Gibson and Friend's perspectives resemble each other in the supposition that in the social construction of a positive identity, oppressed individuals work to make their lives meaningful, and the skills, feelings, and attitudes acquired by many people are resources that facilitate adjustment to aging. However, social workers must be aware of the potential for value judgments affecting professional objectivity when the term "successful aging" is used to refer to subgroups of older adults, and should consider using less value-laden terms in referring to diverse experiences in aging.

Implications of Stoller and Gibson and Friend's perspectives for social work research include the need to develop models of practice interventions with older adults on the micro, mezzo, and macro levels that are sensitive to differences in experiences related to gender, ethnicity, race, sexual orientation, socioeconomic status, and the intersections of these identities for individuals throughout their lifetimes. Researchers need to approach studies of older adults with the understanding that events within socio-historical periods shape the aging experiences of all members of a cohort, but impact differently on disadvantaged and advantaged members. In view of Stoller and Gibson's emphasis on the importance of understanding intersections along multiple hierarchies within individuals, it would also be useful for researchers to explore the intersections of hierarchies within gay men and lesbian women and their implications for identity development and characteristics useful in later adulthood. Expanding the population studied with regard to these issues to include bisexual and transgender persons could also provide important information to social workers planning and providing services to older persons belonging to these groups.

Adaptive resources and meanings created by older adults throughout their lives need to be identified by researchers and validated by social workers providing services. Researchers also need to study whether there have been responses of gay men and lesbian women to heterosexism within various socio-historical periods that have differed from responses proposed by Friend, as well as differences in the effects of responses to heterosexism on adjustment to aging within different cohorts. Studies that identify experiences that contribute to development of coping skills, resilience, and reinforcement of strengths, as well as impediments to developing these characteristics, can contribute new knowledge to develop practice approaches to support the development of strengths useful in later adulthood. We should also study identity development in later adulthood, in addition to earlier years, since we know that changes continue during later adulthood.

REFERENCES

Ashford, J., Lecroy, C., & Lortie, K. (2001). *Human behavior in the social environment: A multidimensional perspective.* Belmont, CA: Wadsworth.

Atchley, R. (1999). *Continuity and adaptation in aging: Creating positive experiences.* Baltimore: The Johns Hopkins University Press.

Atchley, R. (2000). *Social forces and aging: An introduction to social gerontology.* Belmont, CA: Wadsworth.

Austrian, S. (Ed.) (2002). *Developmental theories through the life cycle.* New York: Columbia University Press.

Berger, R. (1982a). The unseen minority: Older gays and lesbians. *Social Work, 27,* 236-242.

Berger, R. (1982b). *Gay and gray.* Urbana: University of Illinois Press.

Berger, R., McBreen, J., & Rifkin, M. (1996). *Human behavior: A perspective for the helping professions.* White Plains, NY: Longman Publishers.

Cass, V. (1979). Homosexual identity formation: A theoretical model. *Journal of homosexuality, 4,* 219-235.

Clark, M., & Anderson, B. (1967). *Culture and aging.* Springfield, IL: Thomas.

Coleman, E. (1981/1982). Developmental stages of the coming out process. *Journal of Homosexuality*, *7*, 31-43.

Council on Social Work Education (2003). *Handbook of accreditation standards and procedures*. Alexandria, VA: Council on Social Work Education.

Council on Social Work Education/*SAGE-SW* (2001). *A blueprint for the new millennium*. Alexandria, VA: Council on Social Work Education.

Fisher, J. (1993). A framework for describing developmental change among older adults. *Adult Education Quarterly*, *43*, 76-89.

Francher, S., & Henkin, J. (1973). The menopausal queen. *American Journal of Orthopsychiatry*, *43*, 670-674.

Friend, R. (1980). GAYging: Adjustment and the older gay male. *Alternative Lifestyles*, *3*, 231-248.

Friend, R. (1991). Older lesbian and gay people: A theory of successful aging, *Journal of Homosexuality*, *20*, 99-118.

Hess, Beth. (1990). Beyond dichotomy: Drawing distinctions and embracing differences. *Sociological Forum*, *5*, 75-93.

Hutchison, E. (2003a). *Dimensions of human behavior: The changing life course*. Thousand Oaks, CA: Pine Forge Press.

Hutchison, E. (2003b). *Dimensions of human behavior: Person and environment*. Thousand Oaks, CA: Pine Forge Press.

Kehoe, M. (1988). Lesbians over 60 speak for themselves, *Journal of Homosexuality*, *16*, 1-111.

Kelly, J. (1977). The aging male homosexual: Myth and reality. *The Gerontologist*, *17*, 328-332.

Kimmel, D. (1978). Adult development and aging: A gay perspective. *Journal of Social Issues*, *34*, 113-130.

Kimmel, D. (1977). Psychotherapy and the older gay man. *Psychotherapy: Theory, Research, and Practice*, *14*, 386-393.

Lee, J. (1997). Going public: A study in the sociology of homosexual liberation. *Journal of Homosexuality*, *3*, 49-78.

Longres, J. (2000). *Human behavior in the social environment*. Itasca, IL: F.E. Peacock Publishers, Inc.

Martin, D., & Lyon, P. (1979). The older lesbian. In B. Berzon & R. Leighton (Eds.), *Positively gay*. Millbrae, CA: Celestial Arts.

Minton, H., & McDonald, G. (1983/1984). Homosexual identity formation as a developmental process. *Journal of Homosexuality*, *9*, 91-104.

Moody, H. (1988). Toward a critical gerontology: The contribution of the humanities to theories of aging. In J. Birren & V. Bengtson (Eds.), *Emergent theories of aging* (pp. 19-40). New York: Springer Publishing Company.

Norlin, J., Chess,W., Dale, O., & Smith, R. (2003). *Human behavior and the social environment: Social systems theory*. Boston: Allyn and Bacon.

Padgett, D. (1999). Aging minority women. In L. Peplau, S. DeBro, R. Veneigas, & P. Taylor (Eds.), *Gender, culture, and ethnicity: Current research about women and men* (pp. 173-181). Mountain View, CA: Mayfield Publishing Company.

Raphael, S., & Robinson, M. (1980). The older lesbian. *Alternative Lifestyles*, *3*, 207-229.

Robbins, S., Chatterjee, P., & Canda, E. (1998). *Contemporary human behavior theory: A critical perspective.* Boston: Allyn and Bacon.

Schriver, J. (2001). *Human behavior and the social environment: Shifting paradigms in essential knowledge for social work practice.* Needham Heights, MA: Allyn and Bacon.

Stoller, E., & Gibson, R. (1997). Advantages of using the life course framework in studying aging. In E. Stoller, & R. Gibson (Eds.), *Worlds of difference: Inequality in the aging experience* (pp. 3-15). Thousand Oaks, CA: Pine Forge Press.

Stoller, E., & Gibson, R. (2000a). Advantages of using the life course framework in studying aging. In E. Stoller, & R. Gibson (Eds.), *Worlds of difference: Inequality in the aging experience* (pp. 19-32). Thousand Oaks, CA: Pine Forge Press.

Stoller, E., & Gibson, R. (2000b). Introduction: Different worlds in aging: Gender, race, and class. In E. Stoller, & R. Gibson (Eds.), *Worlds of difference: Inequality in the aging experience* (pp. 1-15). Thousand Oaks, CA: Pine Forge Press.

Weinberg, M. (1970). The male homosexual: Age-related variations in social and psychological characteristics. *Social Problems, 17,* 527-537.

Zastrow, C., & Kirst-Ashman, K. (2001). *Understanding human behavior and the social environment.* Belmont, CA: Wadsworth.

SPECIAL POPULATIONS

Gay, Lesbian, Bisexual, and Transgender (GLBT) Elders: The Challenges and Resilience of this Marginalized Group

Sandra S. Butler

SUMMARY. Current gay, lesbian, bisexual, and transgender (GLBT) individuals age 65 years and older grew up before the Gay Rights movement. They have learned over many years to hide their identities in order to avoid discrimination and ridicule. Unfortunately, this secrecy has led to the near invisibility of the elder GLBT population and to poor health

Sandra S. Butler, PhD, is Associate Professor, School of Social Work, University of Maine, 5770 Social Work Building, Orono, ME 04469-5770 (E-mail: subtler@maine.edu).

[Haworth co-indexing entry note]: "Gay, Lesbian, Bisexual, and Transgender (GLBT) Elders: The Challenges and Resilience of this Marginalized Group." Butler, Sandra S. Co-published simultaneously in *Journal of Human Behavior in the Social Environment* (The Haworth Social Work Practice Press, an imprint of The Haworth Press, Inc.) Vol. 9, No. 4, 2004, pp. 25-44; and: *Diversity and Aging in the Social Environment* (eds: Sherry M. Cummings, and Colleen Galambos) The Haworth Social Work Practice Press, an imprint of The Haworth Press, Inc., 2004, pp. 25-44. Single or multiple copies of this article are available for a fee from The Haworth Document Delivery Service [1-800-HAWORTH, 9:00 a.m. - 5:00 p.m. (EST). E-mail address: docdelivery@haworthpress.com].

and service access. This paper reviews what we know about GLBT elders, describes some of the unique strengths they bring to the aging process, and outlines some of the challenges they face. Micro, mezzo, and macro practice implications are suggested. *[Article copies available for a fee from The Haworth Document Delivery Service: 1-800-HAWORTH. E-mail address: <docdelivery@haworthpress.com> Website: <http://www. Haworth Press.com> © 2004 by The Haworth Press, Inc. All rights reserved.]*

KEYWORDS. GLBT aging, gay and lesbian elders, homophobia, gay sensitive programs/policies, culturally competent practice

INTRODUCTION

It has been well-documented that health and social service systems are often perceived as unwelcoming by gay, lesbian, bisexual, and transgender (GLBT) individuals. Brotman, Ryan, and Cormier (2003) list some of the negative reactions from service providers which gay men and lesbians encounter: "embarrassment, anxiety, inappropriate reactions, direct rejection of the patient or exhibition of hostility, harassment, excessive curiosity, pity, condescension, ostracism, refusal of treatment, detachment, avoidance of physical contact, or breach of confidentiality" (p. 192). They offer further that discrimination toward lesbians and gay men may be particularly pervasive in the elder care system which has gone largely unchallenged with respect to its treatment of GLBT elders. This article examines the situation of GLBT elders, the strengths they bring to the aging process, and the challenges they face in society and within the health and social service system. It concludes with micro, mezzo and macro practice suggestions for proactively improving the conditions of this marginalized group.

Historical Context

It has only been three decades since the American Psychiatric Association (APA) removed homosexuality from the list of mental disorders discussed in the *Diagnostic and Statistical Manual of Mental Disorders*(DSM). In the first two editions of this manual (DSM-I, 1952 and DSM-II, 1968), homosexuals were labeled as sexual deviants and classified as child molesters, voyeurs, exhibitionists, and people who committed antisocial or destructive crimes (Hidalgo, Peterson, & Woodman, 1985). Fortunately, the struggles for civil rights that swept the country in the 1950s and 1960s created fertile ground for the gay rights movement, a movement that has worked to change society's perception and treatment of gay men, lesbians, and more recently bisexuals and transgender individuals.

It is often said that the gay rights movement began with the Stonewall riots in June 1969, when the New York City Police Department went on a:

> . . . routine assignment to harass patrons and close a gay bar in Green-wich Village. They were unexpectedly faced with the anger and in-dignation of a handful of men and women who felt they had had enough. That night began subsequent rioting and brought gays out of their "closet" around the city. This capped a history of quietly suf-fered oppression. (Kochman, 1997, p. 6)

Many GLBT individuals who are currently 65 years of age or older, were among those who quietly endured this oppression in their younger years; among these elders are the courageous activists who fought to create a more welcoming world for themselves and future GLBT generations to follow.

As a consequence of these efforts, the context has changed since 1969. In 1973, the APA removed homosexuality from its official list of disorders. This action rippled through the helping professions, including the profession of social work. Prior to the APA revision, social work had been guilty of de-fining homosexuality as an illness and subjecting gay clients to conversion (to heterosexuality) treatment (Kochman, 1997). In 1977, the National Asso-ciation of Social Workers (NASW) adopted a policy statement on gay issues which reflected its change of heart:

> NASW views discrimination and prejudice directed against any mi-nority as inimical to the mental health not only of the affected minor-ity, but of the society as a whole. The Association deplores and will work to combat archaic laws, discriminatory employment practices, and other forms of discrimination which serve to impose something less than equal status upon homosexually-oriented members of the human family. (1977 NASW Policy Statement as cited in Hidalgo et al., 1985, p. 162)

SOCIAL WORK POSITIONS TODAY

In the quarter century that has passed since this policy statement was written, social work has remained committed to understanding "the complex issues that lesbian, gay, and bisexual people encounter within the dominant culture in order to provide services respectful of each individual" (NASW, 2000, p. 193). Guided by the *NASW Code of Ethics* (1996), which bans discrimination on the basis of sexual orientation and encourages social workers to expand access, choices and opportunities to marginalized groups, the NASW policy statement in the 5th edition of *Social Work Speaks* (NASW, 2000) reflects the profession's ongoing commitment to improving the lives of gay men, lesbians, and bisexuals. (Interestingly, while bisexuals were added to the policy statement in 2000, transgendered individuals have not yet been included.) The more recent statement begins:

> It is the position of NASW that same-gender sexual orientation should be afforded the same respect and rights as other-gender orientation. Discrimination and prejudice directed against any group are damaging to the social, emotional, and economic well-being of the affected group and of society as a whole. NASW is committed to advancing policies and practices that will improve the status and well-being of all lesbian, gay, and bisexual people. (p. 197)

Furthermore, NASW includes attention to sexual orientation in its policy statement regarding long-term care. It states that long-term care reform should include "access to long-term care services for all who need them, regardless of age, income, disability, race, national origin, gender, sexual orientation, ethnicity, or geographic location" (NASW, 2000, p. 212). Reflecting these policy statements, social work texts and curriculum have increasingly included content on the life situations, experiences of discrimination, and service needs of potential GLBT clients. Nonetheless, perhaps mirroring the ageism within both U.S. society (Hooyman & Kiyak, 2002) and our profession (NASW, 2000), content on GLBT individuals in their later years is less evident.

INVISIBILITY OF GLBT ELDERS

The invisibility of GLBT elders is a function of several factors. GLBT individuals who grew up before the Stonewall riots, "gay liberation," and the removal of homosexuality as a disease in the DSM-III, learned the importance of hiding their identity (Barranti & Cohen, 2000; Connolly, 1996; McLeod, 1997). "This cohort when they were young was labeled sick by doctors, immoral by clergy, unfit by the military, and a menace by the police" (Kochman, 1997, p. 2). Thus, elder GLBT have become very practiced at concealment. In their youth and young adulthood, they learned to hide their orientation from family, friends and employers; some chose heterosexual marriage and having children as one way to conceal their sexual orientation from society–and maybe themselves (D'Augelli, Grossman, Hershberger, & O'Connell, 2001; Sitter, 1997). Blando (2001) refers to elder lesbians and gay men as "twice hidden" and the most "invisible of an already invisible minority" (p. 87). It is important to note, however, that some portion of today's elder GLBT have come out in their middle-age, and that their experiences may be different from those who identified as GLBT in their youth, during the more oppressive pre-liberation years.

While society may be somewhat more welcoming to GLBT individuals than it was 30 years ago, heterosexism remains pervasive and homophobia has not disappeared. Heterosexism can be defined as an ideological system that denies, denigrates and stigmatizes any non-heterosexual form of behavior, identity, relationship or community (Cahill, South, & Spade, 2000); heterosexism refers to beliefs and attitudes that favor opposite-sex over same-sex partnerships (Van Wormer, Wells, & Boes, 2000). Homophobia is the irrational fear of homosexuals and the hatred of GLB individuals based solely on their sexual orientation (Cahill et al., Kochman, 1997; Van Wormer et al.). Social prejudice against transgendered people, also known as transphobia, can be, in many cases, even more intense than that directed against lesbians and gay men (Cook-Daniels, 1997).

In most parts of the United States (though selected cities, states, and businesses have nondiscrimination ordinances, laws and clauses), it is legal to discriminate against GLBT people in housing, employment and basic civil rights. In 16 states, archaic sodomy laws continue to brand GLBT individuals as criminal despite ongoing efforts to repeal these statutes (Meyer, 2001). The recent Supreme Court decision, Lawrence et al. v. Texas, June 26, 2003, invalidates the sodomy laws in Texas and is expected to impact enforcement of such laws in other states as well. Notwithstanding this recent victory, it is not only understandable, but even prudent for elder GLBT to remain cautious about "coming out," i.e., disclosing their sexual orientation.

In addition to the heterosexism, homophobia, and transphobia that affect GLBT individuals across their lifespan, ageism is an added insult for the GLBT elder. The GLBT community has not been immune to the youth worship reflected in mainstream U.S. society (Connolly, 1996; Van Wormer et al., 2000). Gay culture has been guilty of being particularly youth focused; what is old has been seen as less attractive and less worthy than what is young (Brotman et al. 2003). "Manifestations of ageism within the GLBT community include beauty standards that privilege youth, the exclusion of old people from community discussions, and the absence of senior issues from the mainstream GLBT agenda" (Cahill et al., 2000, p. 18).

WHO ARE GLBT ELDERS?

While there has been increasing research on GLBT elders in recent years, what we know is gathered from relatively few studies, which are based on small non-representative samples. As the editor of a special issue of the *American Journal of Public Health* devoted to GLBT health issues, Meyer (2001) notes that there are obstacles which stand "in the way of our gathering knowledge about LGBT [a variation on the acronym used in this article] populations. Some methodological; others are related to homophobia and heterosexism, which place LGBT studies outside the mainstream in terms of importance and allocation of resources" (p. 857).

In the seminal report, *Outing Age: Public Policy Issues Affecting Gay, Lesbian, Bisexual and Transgender Elders*, published by the Policy Institute of the National Gay and Lesbian Task Force in 2000, Cahill and his co-authors synthesize current research–as meager as it is–in a section titled, "What Do We Know About GLBT Elders?" They begin by documenting the limitations of research in the field to date. Most studies are of gay men, with a smaller number on lesbians, and very few which include bisexual or transgender individuals. Furthermore, most of the studies utilized small samples that do not reflect the racial and economic diversity within the GLBT community (Cahill et al., 2000; Christian & Keefe, 1997). While not always easily gleaned from existing research, GLBT elders vary in socio-demographic characteristics such as culture, ethnic, or racial identity; physical ability; income; education; and place of residence. "They are also diverse in the degree to which their LGBT identities are central to their self-definition, their level of affiliation with other LGBT people, and their rejection or acceptance of societal stereotypes and prejudice" (Meyer, 2001, p. 856). Herdt, Beeler, and Rawls (1997) reiterate the limitations of our current state of knowledge:

> [I]n the case of older bisexuals, lesbians and gays, the combination of poor research literature, clinical samples, and dated historical narratives from prior generations has had the effect of making this

population appear more homogeneous than it is, undercutting diversity in life-course experiences. (p. 234)

With these caveats in mind, what do we know about this population of elders? It is difficult to be precise when estimating the number of GLBT seniors. Only recently have there been beginning efforts to estimate the number of transgender individuals in the United States–individuals who fall along the full range of sexual orientation from homosexual to bisexual to heterosexual, and into many subcategories based on numerous factors (Witten, 2002)–thus, transgender individuals are not included in the following estimates. Conservative estimates of the prevalence of gay men, lesbians and bisexuals in the U.S. population range from 3% to 8%; this is likely to be an undercount due to the ongoing taboo of identifying as gay, lesbian or bisexual in an interview or survey (Cahill et al., 2000). Using this estimated prevalence rate, Cahill, South and Spade suggest that there are currently from 1 million to 2.8 million GLB individuals aged 65 or older, and, based on Administration on Aging estimates of elder population growth, they predict that this number will increase to 2 to 6 million by 2030. The population of GLBT elders includes the same racial and class diversity as the larger U.S. population. Despite a widespread myth that gay men and lesbians are economically privileged, multiple studies have shown this not to be the case at all. Anti-gay activists and government officials, including Supreme Court Justice Scalia, have portrayed gays and lesbians as wealthy in order to justify opposing non-discrimination laws (Cahill et al., 2000).

Based on limited research, it appears that elder GLBT individuals are more likely to live alone than their heterosexual counterparts. They are also less likely to be living with life partners and less likely to have children than heterosexual seniors (Cahill et al., 2000). For example, one New York City-based study found 65% of their sample of 253 gay and lesbian seniors to live alone; this was nearly twice the rate of living alone among the entire population of New Yorkers 65 and older (36%) (Brookdale Center, 1999). Another study with a sample of gay and lesbian elders in the Los Angeles area found that 75% of their respondents reported living alone (Rosenfeld, 1999).

It is important to distinguish living alone from being lonely. There is a pervasive stereotype of GLBT elders as lonely and isolated. This caricature has been refuted repeatedly in the literature (Blando, 2001; Christian & Keefe, 1997; Whitford, 1997): GLBT elders are no more lonely than heterosexual elders or than GLBT younger adults (Cahill et al., 2000). Moreover, some have posited that GLBT elders may have a social advantage given their well-developed social networks of choice, often relying less on family and/or spouses, which provide a broad base of support in times of loss and need (Barranti & Cohen, 2000; Butler & Hope, 1999; Healy, 2002). Committed partner relationships are important to many GLBT elders; surveys of gay and lesbian individuals have documented "a range of 40-60% of gay men and 45-80% of lesbians in a committed relationship at any given time" (Cahill et al., 2000, p. 10). One study specifically of elder gays and lesbians in Chicago found 79% of lesbians were partnered as were 46% of gay men (Herdt et al., 1997).

STRENGTH GLBT INDIVIDUALS BRING TO THE AGING PROCESS

While it can be argued that there is a great deal of similarity in the aging process across lines of gender and sexual orientation, it is useful to outline some of the distinctive situations and experiences that may impact GLBT elders. Contrary to the myths of a pathetic and lonely old age, many gay men and lesbians approach their elder years with unique resiliency and particular strengths (Butler & Hope, 1999; Healy, 2002; Van Wormer et al., 2000). Barranti and Cohen (2000) enumerate specific factors which may allow GLBT individuals to enter their elder years with greater ease than their non-GLBT peers:

- Coping skills developed through the process of accepting their sexual identity may help GLBT seniors in the acceptance of aging.
- Skills developed through the coming out process and the management of the social perception of "difference" throughout life prepare GLBT individuals for society's perception of older people in a youth-oriented society.
- The stigma of being older is often experienced as less severe than the stigma of being "queer," which gay men and lesbians faced in their youth.
- In part due to rejections by families of origin and/or procreation, GLBT individuals often create "families of choice," which are able to provide extensive social support in times of need.
- Greater flexibility in gender roles exhibited by GLBT individuals can be helpful in the aging process.

Despite these advantages, gay and lesbian people do experience some obstacles in their latter years not shared with their heterosexual cohorts. While there is greater acceptance of gay and lesbian relationships and GLBT individuals in general in our society than existed 30 years ago, considerable discrimination, stigma, and overt hatred toward homosexuality remain (Brotman et al., 2003). For safety and economic reasons, many GLBT older adults have been required to lead their entire lives "in the closet"; often their sexual orientation becomes even more invisible with age.

SPECIFIC CHALLENGES FACED BY GLBT ELDERS

Heterosexism, homophobia, transphobia, legal discrimination, and the inability of GLBT partners to benefit from the advantages of being married spouses lead to many specific problems and barriers to service for GLBT seniors (Smith & Calvert, 2001). I will enumerate a few of these challenges here, drawing largely from the work of Cahill, South, and Spade (2000); for a more comprehensive discussion of these issues, see the full *Outing Age* report (Cahill et al.).

Access to services. There are a very small number of organizations whose mission is specifically to meet the needs of GLBT elders. They exist in large cities with relatively visible GLBT communities. The largest of these is Senior Action in a Gay Environment (SAGE), located in New York City, with satellite programs in numerous other cities in the United States and Canada. Gay and Lesbian Outreach to Elders (GLOE), a program of New Leaf: Services to Our Community, is another GLBT elder organization, which is located in San Francisco. A small volunteer organization, Senior Health Resources, has recently been initiated in Washington D.C. to serve elder GLBT individuals. Notwithstanding these metropolitan areas, the majority of GLBT elders in the country do not have access to such specialized services and must seek services in more mainstream aging organizations such as the Area Agencies on Aging (AAAs).

Most mainstream aging organizations are not sensitive to the needs of GLBT elders. For example, a 1994 study of 24 AAAs found that 96% did not offer any services specifically designed for GLBT elders, nor did they target outreach efforts to the GLBT community. Lesbian and gay elders who lived in the regions served by these AAAs confirmed through a companion survey that AAAs had a long way to go in terms of providing services to gay and lesbian seniors (Behney, 1994).

The British publication, *Opening Doors: Working with Older Lesbians and Gay Men* (Smith & Calvert, 2001), challenges service organizations to create an environment of positive acceptance and welcome for lesbian and gay clients, as well as for their lesbian and gay staff and volunteers. The authors present numerous myths which often prevent mainstream service agencies from providing gay-sensitive services or doing outreach to the GLBT elder community (pp. 8-10); three of these are described below.

One myth frequently stated by service organizations when challenged to be accessible to GLBT individuals is: "there aren't any around here." The veracity of such statements is highly unlikely as GLBT individuals are everywhere and they are a diverse population. The majority of elder GLBT do not conform to society's stereotypes of effeminate gay men and masculine lesbians; after all, many of them have spent a lifetime trying to pass as heterosexual. Agencies serving older adults should assume that at least 5%, or one in 20, of the clients they serve are gay, lesbian, bisexual, or transgender.

A second common myth is "we're open to everyone anyway." As with any marginalized group, a passive open-door, "color-blind" approach may not be adequate to make services appear safe to elder GLBT. In order for an organization to meet the needs of any minority group, it needs to understand the nature of those needs.

> Equally important is the need for an organization to demonstrate its inclusiveness. After the centuries of intolerance displayed towards lesbians and gay men, it is entirely reasonable that they might assume an organization to be indifferent or even hostile until it proves itself otherwise. (Smith & Calvert, 2001, p. 9)

A third myth listed by Smith and Calvert (2001) is "no one has ever asked, so there is obviously no need" (p. 9). As discussed earlier, most members of the current cohort of GLBT elders lived much of their lives outside what society has considered acceptable. Younger GLBT individuals, who have grown up post gay-liberation and who have been "out," or public about their sexual orientation, may be more likely to demand appropriate services than current GLBT elders. Without a collective voice to represent them, it is unlikely that older GLBT clients will "take any initiative which might bring to light their sexual orientation until an agency has shown it is ready to listen sympathetically" (Smith & Calvert, p. 9). In other words, agencies need to be proactive in their efforts to be accessible, to feel safe, and to serve the needs of older GLBT individuals.

In order for service agencies to "open their doors" and to become an accepting and safe place for elder GLBT clients, they will need to confront these myths and proactively change some of their practices. Smith and Calvert (2001) provide several examples of mainstream agencies serving older adults in England (called Age Concern agencies) that have begun the work of opening their doors to older gay men and lesbians. Two of their examples follow:

> Age Concern Gloucester has taken part in training sessions and is expanding services to older lesbians and gay men. Its leaflets and promotional material state the Organization recognizes [sic] the needs of older lesbians and gay people, without singling them out. (p. 17)

> Age Concern Nottingham and Nottinghamshire forged working links with a local organization called OUTHOUSE in 1999. OUTHOUSE will eventually be a community center for older lesbian and gay people. It will include rooms that Age Concern can use; e.g., [sic] for information and advice sessions. Meanwhile, Age Concern and OUTHOUSE are maintaining close relations and cross referring users as appropriate. (p. 26)

Making aging services more accessible to GLBT elders is not unlike making services more welcoming for racial and ethnic minorities and other oppressed groups: it is challenging, but getting it right is rewarding.

Lack of recognition of GLBT families. Legal marriage affords certain rights and privileges which are unavailable to same-sex partners. People of the same sex are not allowed to marry and domestic partnerships are neither widely available nor as comprehensive as the rights and responsibilities of marriage (Cahill et al., 2000). Some rights unavailable to GLBT partners include Social Security benefits for survivors, employee health benefits, inheritance, housing and hospital visitation.

> GLBT people encounter these issues specifically as they age because they may rely more and more on families to provide care or make critical decisions. This frequently places GLBT people in a position where their blood relatives have more power to make im-

portant decisions for them than their partners who are not related by blood or law. (Cahill et al., p. 43)

Cahill and his co-authors suggest that Social Security's treatment of same-sex couples may be the most blatant and costly example of institutionalized heterosexism in federal policy. Under the current Social Security system, married spouses, some divorced spouses, and children are eligible for survivor benefits; unmarried spouses (e.g., same-sex partners) are ineligible for these benefits no matter how many years they may have lived with and supported their partners. Similarly, minor children in unrecognized GLBT families are ineligible for benefits (Dubois, 1999). The Social Security Administration estimated that in 1998, 781,000 widows and widowers received an average of $442 a month in survivor benefits, costing the Social Security system $4.1 billion (Cahill et al., 2000). If only 3% of those individuals who survived their life partners were gay or lesbian, the failure to pay Social Security benefits to GLBT surviving partners would total about $124 million a year (Cahill et al., 2000).

The spousal benefit in Social Security is also unavailable to same-sex couples. While less important to partners with relatively equal incomes, the spousal benefit is helpful to married couples in which one spouse has a higher income. The spouse with lower earnings can choose to receive the Social Security monthly benefit based on his or her own work history or one-half the monthly benefit to which the other spouse is entitled based on his or her own work history. Cahill, South and Spade (2000) provide an example of how the spousal and survivor benefits can impact same-sex couples with unequal earnings.

... Frank and Stella are a legally married couple who have been together for 40 years. At age 65 Stella, who was the main breadwinner for the couple, is entitled to a monthly Social Security benefit of $1,400. Frank is entitled to a monthly benefit for $500 based on his own work history. Under the spousal benefit option, Frank can choose to receive $700 a month, or half of Stella's monthly benefit, instead of the $500 he would receive based on his own work history. Thus due to the spousal benefit, Frank is entitled to an additional $200 a month, or $2400 a year. Now assume Stanley and Juan are a gay male couple who have supported each other for 40 years. Juan receives $1,400 a month, while Stanley receives only $500. Stanley is ineligible for the spousal benefit, which would be $700 a month if Juan were Stanley's wife instead of his male partner; thus Stanley loses out on $200 a month, or $2,400 a year. (p. 44)

Lack of recognition for same-sex partners also negatively affects GLBT elders' access to pensions, 401(k) plans, and disability benefits. (See Cahill et al., [2000] for more detail.) Access to these benefits would contribute greatly to the quality of life for many GLBT elders–particularly those with low incomes.

> Even if some jurisdictions allow marriage by same gender couples in the near future, the availability of federal benefits such as Social Security benefits will continue to be available only to heterosexual, traditional families under the current provisions of the Defense of Marriage Act as passed by Congress in 1996. (Dubois, 1999, pp. 290-291)

> While the long-term goal for policy change is to amend Social Security regulations so that the surviving partner of the same-sex couple can receive benefits just as married widows and widowers do and to ensure equal treatment of same-sex spouses under the spousal benefit provisions, this change is unlikely in the near future. For some GLBT elders, seeking legal assistance in their long-term financial and health care planning from a gay-friendly attorney can ameliorate this unequal situation. (Dubois, 1999)

The phenomenon of "Medicaid spend down," which is traumatic for any elder, has particular significance for GLBT elders. Nursing home care is very costly; Medicare covers only short-term acute care (no more than 100 days) in nursing facilities (Hooyman & Kiyak, 2002). Individuals needing long-term care must either privately pay for nursing home care, have long-term care insurance (which may not be comprehensive), or rely on Medicaid once all other assets have been depleted (i.e., the Medicaid spend down). Income and asset protections have been put in place to protect the impoverishment of spouses of heterosexual nursing home residents using Medicaid. For example, these legally married spouses may remain in their homes until death, before the state may attempt to recover some of the costs of care through an estate recovery process (Cahill et al., 2000); this is not available to the same-sex partner of a nursing home resident (Dubois, 1999), potentially leading to homelessness for a life-long partner whose loved one has become ill. "This unequal treatment can force same-sex couples into a Hobson's choice between getting the medical coverage to meet a partner's health care needs or foregoing medical care in order to avoid giving up the couple's home and life savings" (Cahill, 2002, p. 8).

On the other hand, GLBT partners do have one advantage over married spouses who require Medicaid for long-term care. The married spouse of a nursing home resident must also spend down his or her assets to a federally-set limit, something that would not be legally mandated for an unmarried partner (Dubois, 1999). For example, in Washington state, as of August 1, 2003, the permissible assets for the married spouse of a Medicaid-financed nursing home resident will be reduced from $90,660 to $40,000 (National Center, 2003). (The community-living spouse may also keep his or her house, car, and certain other necessities.) This mandated limit on a spouse's assets does not apply to unmarried partners, something that would be helpful to GLBT partners who have significant assets. However, the less well-off GLBT elder whose partner requires Medicaid-financed, long-term care has no legal protection regarding their shared home or other assets.

Nursing homes and homophobia. While less than 5% of older adults over 65 reside in nursing homes at any one time (Hooyman & Kiyak, 2002), the fear of ending one's life in a nursing facility is pervasive. This fear is particularly ubiquitous among GLBT elders who worry that their integrity and life choices will not be honored as they become physically frail and/or mentally vulnerable (Butler & Hope, 1999; Connolly, 1996; Quam, 1997). When GLBT elders enter mainstream assisted living, nursing facilities, or retirement communities, they are frequently presumed to be heterosexual; their long-term partnerships may not be recognized or valued. "Even if they had lived openly in the past, they may suddenly find themselves in situations where disclosing their sexual orientation or gender variance makes them vulnerable to discrimination or even abuse" (Cahill et al., 2000, p. 53).

Cook-Daniels (1997) provides two examples of homophobic abuse of frail GLBT elders. In one case, nursing home staff refused to bathe an elder resident because they did not want to touch "the lesbian." In another instance a home care assistant threatened to "out" (i.e., reveal his sexual orientation) her elder gay male client if he reported her negligent care. Another example, illustrating both how society desexualizes older people and the compounding influence of homophobia, is provided by Cahill (2002):

. . . a nursing assistant entered a room in a nursing facility without knocking and saw two elderly male residents engaging in oral sex. The two were separated immediately after the assistant notified her supervisor. Within a day, one man was transferred to a psychiatric ward and placed in four point restraints. A community health board held that the transfer was a warranted response to "deviant behavior." (p. 6)

A study of social worker perceptions of staff attitudes in 29 different nursing homes in New York State revealed a high level of homophobia and heterosexism among long-term care staff (Fairchild, Carrino, & Ramirez, 1996). Most of the social workers in this study said the staff at their nursing homes were intolerant or condemning of homosexuality; over a third of the sample avoided the question about attitudes toward homosexuality altogether, perhaps revealing a significant level of homophobia among the social workers themselves. All but three social workers described staff attitudes toward homosexuality as negative, using terms such as: "horrendous," "frightened," "more uncomfortable," "horrified," "anger," and "gross." Only one social worker out of the 29 thought staff would be tolerant and just two others stated that attitudes would be a mix of tolerance and intolerance. One social worker described how her nursing home tries to avoid the whole issue of gay and lesbian residents by making it a part of admission policy to forbid partners of the same sex to move into the facility (Fairchild et al.). Clearly, there is ample foundation for the fears GLBT elders have concerning their treatment, should they find themselves in a nursing home at some point in their lives.

Brotman, Ryan, and Cormier (2003) have suggested that if the issue of sexuality in general is made more open in elder care sectors, then sexual orientation is more likely to be addressed. Ageism has reinforced the perception that sex is only for the young and repressive attitudes have contributed to making sexuality a feared topic in elder care settings. Brotman et al., suggest that broad organizational change in this area will likely benefit the elder GLBT individual. Promoting discussion of sexuality in general in the organizational setting, which has traditionally placed little significance on privacy and discouraged sexual activity, may increase openness to the issues and needs of GLBT residents.

PRACTICE AND POLICY IMPLICATIONS

Given the strengths that GLBT elders bring to the aging process as well as the extra challenges they face in our heterosexist, homophobic and transphobic society, there are implications for both culturally competent practice and proactive policy change. In order to lessen and eventually eliminate both the subtle and blatant discrimination and oppression faced by current and future GLBT seniors, attention must be paid to micro, mezzo, and macro level practice. I will outline some suggestions on where we can begin.

Micro level practice. Healy (2002) offers a guide for culturally competent practice with elder lesbian families which can be adapted to address the needs of all GLBT elders. Healy suggests that practitioners increase their awareness by engaging in self-reflection regarding their own views pertaining to sexual orientation and gender identity. Just as practitioners need to recognize their own racism and do anti-racist work in order to work more effectively with clients of differing races and ethnicities, so must they examine their internalized homophobia, heterosexism and prejudices regarding gender identity before working with GLBT clients.

Another suggestion for culturally competent practice offered by Healy (2002) is to question one's assumptions about sexual orientation. Practitioners should not assume they know the sexual orientation or gender identity of their clients, nor the gender of their clients' partners. By resisting these assumptions, practitioners will be more open to understanding the experiences and needs of their clients. For example, it is important to avoid gendered pronouns when asking about significant others; rather, practitioners should ask their clients if there has been anyone who has been a confidant or who has been very important in their lives.

Culturally competent practice depends on knowledge. Practitioners should expand their knowledge of GLBT friendly resources so that they can refer appropriately. Gaining an understanding of how GLBT elders are treated by public policies and an awareness of legal protections such as wills, health proxies, and durable powers of attorney, will allow the practitioner to be more effective in her or his work with older GLBT clients.

Mezzo and macro level practice. In order to address the particular issues raised in this article, several areas for policy advocacy can be suggested. In terms of access to services, the Older American Act, which authorizes and funds AAAs, would be one policy to target. Cahill et al. (2000) suggest that "language should be added that specifically authorizes outreach to GLBT seniors, along with other underrepresented and underserved populations" (p. 71). The authors caution that such language would need to be accompanied by additional resources so that "funds are not taken away from one needy community and redirected to another" (p. 71), creating counter-productive and needless competition among aging groups. Other suggestions for the AAAs include: asking about sexual orientation, gender identity, and significant relationships in the initial client assessment; offering in-service staff training conducted by GLBT elders; developing outreach strategies in collaboration with local GLBT activists; and developing collaborations with GLBT social service organizations (Cahill et al.).

While it seems unlikely in the current politically conservative climate of the United States, one policy change which would have a dramatic impact on the financial well-being of many GLBT seniors would be to amend Social Security regulations so as to allow the surviving partner of a same-sex couple to receive benefits just as heterosexual married widows and widowers do. Similarly, Medicaid spend-down protections should be amended to include the same-sex partners of individuals who enter nursing homes, so that the community-living partner is able to remain in the couple's home until his or her death without jeopardizing his or her loved one's right to Medicaid coverage (Cahill et al., 2000).

Bringing GLBT sensitive services to elders in long-term care is clearly fertile ground for social work advocacy. Diversity training for staff of nursing homes, assisted living centers, congregate housing and home health care is critical given the documented incidence of heterosexism, homophobia and transphobia in long-term care. Moreover, nursing homes should include detailed sexuality policies and accommodate the appropriate private expression of sexual needs of residents, be they homosexual, bisexual or heterosexual. "The right to privacy is already included in most nursing home regulations, but is not always protected for GLBT seniors" (Cahill et al., 2000, p. 74).

There are ongoing efforts by GLBT aging advocates to confront the heterosexism and homophobia in current policies and programs. One example of a recent success took place with the Joint Commission of Healthcare Organizations (JCAHO); in 2003, JCAHO added respect for "residents' habits and pattern of living (including lifestyle choices related to sexual orientation)" to the requirements in the accreditation manual for assisted living facilities (American Society on Aging [ASA], 2003, p. 3). This policy change is a result of several years of advocacy by organizations such as the ASA's Lesbian and Gay Aging Issues Network (LGAIN) and New York City's SAGE.

Another exciting initiative currently being implemented by SAGE is the National Needs Assessment and Technical Assistance Audit. With funding from the Gill Foundation, AARP Andrus Foundation, Lily Auchincloss Foundation and individual donors, this project seeks to gauge the current level of services for GLBT elders throughout the country; to assess the current level of understanding about GLBT aging concerns among those working with the elderly; and to obtain guidance regarding future directions for the GLBT aging movement in policy and program development (Plumb, 2003). This project has included in-depth phone interviews with key informants, town hall meetings in five locations around the country, an on-line survey, and a focus group on transgender aging issues. Results from this study are currently being analyzed and should contribute significantly to the national dialogue on how best to meet the needs of our GLBT elders.

Today's GLBT elders have lived through years of legalized oppression and discrimination. While their numbers are significant, they are not always visible, having spent many years protecting their private lives, sexual orientation and/or gender identity from public view. Advocacy at the micro, mezzo and macro levels is necessary in order to improve the quality of life for GLBT individuals in their latter years. We've come a long way, but the fight is not over yet.

REFERENCES

American Society on Aging (ASA) (2003, March 3). Assisted living standards to recognize sexual orientation. *ASA Connection: Public Policy Link*–e-newsletter for members of ASA. http://www.asaaging.org/asaconnection.

Barranti, C.C.R., & Cohen, H.L. (2000). Lesbian and gay elders: An invisible minority. In R.L. Schneider, N.P. Kropf, & A.J. Kisor (Eds.), *Gerontological social work: Knowledge, service settings, and special populations* (2nd ed., pp. 343-367). Pacific Grove, CA: Brooks/Cole.

Behney, R. (1994, Winter). The aging network's response to gay and lesbian issues. *Outword: Newsletter of the Lesbian and Gay Aging Issues Network, 1*(2), 2.

Blando, J.A. (2001). Twice hidden: Older gay and lesbian couples, friends, and intimacy. *Generations, 25*(2), 87-89.

Brookdale Center on Aging of Hunter College, & Senior Action in a Gay Environment (SAGE) (1999). *Assistive housing for elderly gays and lesbians in New York City: Extent of need and the preferences of elderly gays and lesbians.* New York: Hunter College and SAGE.

Brotman, S., Ryan, B., & Cormier, R. (2003). The health and social service needs of gay and lesbian elders and their families in Canada. *The Gerontologist, 43*(2), 192-202.

Butler, S.S., & Hope, B. (1999). Health and well-being for late middle-aged and old lesbians in a rural area. *Journal of Gay & Lesbian Social Services, 9*(4), 27-46.

Cahill, S. (2002). Long term care issues affecting gay, lesbian, bisexual and transgender elders. *Geriatric Care Management Journal, 12*(3), 4-8.

Cahill, S., South, K., & Spade, J. (2000). *Outing age: Public policy issues affecting gay, lesbian, bisexual and transgender elders.* Washington, DC: Policy Institute, National Gay and Lesbian Task Force.

Christian, D.V., & Keefe, D.A. (1997). Maturing gay men: A framework for social service assessment and intervention. In J.K. Quam (Ed.), *Social services for senior gay men and lesbians* (pp. 47-78). New York: Harrington Park Press.

Connolly, L. (1996). Long-term care and hospice: The special needs of older gay men and lesbians. *Journal of Gay & Lesbian Social Services, 5*(1), 77-91.

Cook-Daniels, L. (1997). Lesbian, gay male, bisexual and transgendered elders: Elder abuse and neglect issues. *Journal of Elder Abuse & Neglect, 9*(2), 35-49.

D'Augelli, A.R., Grossman, A.H., Hershberger, S.L., & O'Connell, T.S. (2001). Aspects of mental health among older lesbian, gay and bisexual adults. *Aging & Mental Health, 5*(2), 149-158.

Dubois, M.R. (1999). Legal planning for gay, lesbian, and non-traditional elders. *Albany Law Review, 63*(1), 263-332.

Fairchild, S.K., Carrino, G.E., & Ramirez, M. (1996). Social workers' perceptions of staff attitudes toward resident sexuality in a random sample of New York State nursing homes: A pilot study. *Journal of Gerontological Social Work, 26*(1/2), 153-169.

Healy, T. (2002). Culturally competent practice with elderly lesbians. *Geriatric Care Management Journal, 12*(3), 9-13.

Herdt, G., Beeler, J., & Rawls, T.W. (1997). Life course diversity among older lesbians and gay men: A study in Chicago. *Journal of Gay, Lesbian, and Bisexual Identity, 2*(3/4), 231-246.

Hidalgo, H., Peterson, T.L., & Woodman, N.J. (1985). Introduction. In H. Hidalgo, T.L. Peterson, & N.J. Woodman (Eds.), *Lesbian and gay issues: A resource manual for social workers* (pp. 1-6). Silver Spring, MD: NASW, Inc.

Hooyman, N.R., & Kiyak. H.A. (2002). *Social gerontology: A multidisciplinary perspective* (6th ed.). Boston: Allyn and Bacon.

Kochman, A. (1997). Gay and lesbian elderly: Historical overview and implications for social work practice. In J.K. Quam (Ed.), *Social services for senior gay men and lesbians* (pp. 1-10). New York: Harrington Park Press.

McLeod, B. (1997). Yvonne and Helen: Finding a way to trust. In J.K. Quam (Ed.), *Social services for senior gay men and lesbians* (pp. 105-107). New York: Harrington Park Press.

Meyer, I.H. (2001). Why lesbian, gay, bisexual, transgender public health? *American Journal of Public Health, 91*(6), 856-859.

NASW (1996). *NASW code of ethics.* Washington, DC: Author.

National Association of Social Workers (NASW) (2000). *Social work speaks: National Association of Social Workers policy statement 2000-2003* (5th ed.). Washington, DC: Author.

National Center on Caregivers (2003, July 16). *Family Caregiver Alliance Caregiver Policy Digest, 3*(13). Can be retrieved from http:www.caregiving.org/pd.

Plumb, M.(2003, March 10). *National needs assessment and technical assistance audit.* Draft report prepared for Senior Action in a Gay Environment (SAGE). New York: SAGE.

Quam, J.K. (1997). The story of Carrie and Anne: Long-term care crisis. In J.K. Quam (Ed.), *Social services for senior gay men and lesbians* (pp. 97-99). New York: Harrington Park Press.

Rosenfeld, D. (1999). Identity work among lesbian and gay elderly. *Journal of Aging Studies, 13*(2), 121-144.

Sitter, K. (1997). Jim: Coming out at age sixty-two. In J.K. Quam (Ed.), *Social services for senior gay men and lesbians* (pp. 101-104). New York: Harrington Park Press.

Smith, H., & Calvert, J. (2001). *Opening doors: Working with older lesbians and gay men.* London: Aging Concern England.

Van Wormer, K., Wells, J., & Boes, M. (2000). *Social work with lesbians, gays and bisexuals: A strengths perspective.* Boston: Allyn and Bacon.

Whitford, G.S. (1997). Realities and hopes for older gay men. In J.K. Quam (Ed.), *Social services for senior gay men and lesbians* (pp. 79-95). New York: Harrington Park Press.

Witten, T.M. (2002). Geriatric care and management issues for the transgender and intersex populations. *Geriatric Care Management Journal, 12*(3), 20-24.

HIV/AIDS and Aging:
A Diverse Population
of Vulnerable Older Adults

Charles A. Emlet

SUMMARY. Older adults, those age 50 and over, have continually represented approximately 10-15% of all cases of AIDS reported to the Centers for Disease Control and Prevention. In addition to those infected with HIV, many older adult caregivers are affected by HIV/AIDS. Despite these figures, social workers and other providers of health care are often unaware of the needs of these growing populations. Older adults with HIV/AIDS as well as those affected by the disease represent diverse backgrounds in gender, ethnicity, sexual orientation, and exposure to HIV. Additionally, older adults present special issues and challenges not always present in younger individuals with HIV/AIDS. *[Article copies available for a fee from The Haworth Document Delivery Service: 1-800-HAWORTH. E-mail address: <docdelivery@haworthpress.com> Website: <http://www. HaworthPress.com> © 2004 by The Haworth Press, Inc. All rights reserved.]*

Charles A. Emlet, PhD, MSW, is Associate Professor of Social Work, Hartford Geriatric Social Work Faculty Scholar, University of Washington-Tacoma, 1900 Commerce Street, Campus Box 358425, Tacoma, WA 98402 (E-mail: caemlet@u.washington.edu).

The author wishes to acknowledge the support of the John A. Hartford Foundation and the Hartford Geriatric Social Work Faculty Scholars Program in preparing this manuscript.

[Haworth co-indexing entry note]: "HIV/AIDS and Aging: A Diverse Population of Vulnerable Older Adults." Emlet, Charles A. Co-published simultaneously in *Journal of Human Behavior in the Social Environment* (The Haworth Social Work Practice Press, an imprint of The Haworth Press, Inc.) Vol. 9, No. 4, 2004, pp. 45-63; and: *Diversity and Aging in the Social Environment* (eds: Sherry M. Cummings, and Colleen Galambos) The Haworth Social Work Practice Press, an imprint of The Haworth Press, Inc., 2004, pp. 45-63. Single or multiple copies of this article are available for a fee from The Haworth Document Delivery Service [1-800-HAWORTH, 9:00 a.m. - 5:00 p.m. (EST). E-mail address: docdelivery@haworthpress.com].

45

KEYWORDS. Aging, older adults, older persons, HIV/AIDS, HIV disease, vulnerable populations, diversity, social work

Older adults, often defined in HIV research as those age 50 years and over, are increasingly recognized as being at-risk for HIV disease. HIV/AIDS has traditionally been seen as a disease of younger persons. Thus, older adults with HIV/AIDS have been called a *hidden population* (Emlet, 1997) and the *invisible ten percent* (Genke, 2000), referring to the fact that approximately 10% of AIDS cases in the United States have been diagnosed in persons age 50 and over. Although social workers and other health professionals are becoming increasingly aware of the impact HIV/AIDS has on older adults, many stereotypes and ageist attitudes continue to exist. A common myth, for example, is that older adults are not at risk for HIV/AIDS because they are not sexually active. Other stereotypes reinforce beliefs that older adults do not contract HIV from injection drug use or that all older, married couples live in monogamous relationships. Such beliefs create barriers to effective prevention, education, identification, and treatment of HIV disease in older persons.

The purpose of this paper is to educate the reader to the diversity that exists within this emerging population of infected and affected elders. Like older adults in general, those infected with or affected by HIV disease are not a homogeneous group. Various aspects of diversity–including gender, ethnicity, and sexual orientation–as well as differences in risk factors, medical needs, and psychosocial factors are explored. The discussion will conclude by examining older caregivers of persons living with HIV/AIDS, also referred to as being *HIV-affected*.

DEMOGRAPHICS

Although HIV disease has been viewed as affecting those in young adulthood and early middle age (Riley, 1989), individuals over age 50 with AIDS have been consistently reported over the course of the pandemic (Ory & Mack, 1998). Throughout the tracking of AIDS cases by the Centers for Disease Control and Prevention (CDC), 10 to 12% of all diagnosed cases of AIDS in the U.S. have been in those ages 50 and over, translating to 90,513 AIDS cases as of December 2001 (CDC, 2002). This figure does not include older adults diagnosed with HIV (not yet AIDS) or those who received an AIDS diagnosis prior to age 50 and have "aged in" with the disease. According to Wooten-Bielski

(1999), these figures may also underrepresent the actual number of AIDS cases among older persons, as HIV/AIDS goes undiagnosed in older people to a larger degree than in their younger counterparts. Because of the lack of accurate diagnosis, it is possible that many infected older adults die without having been properly diagnosed (Szirony, 1999). Ory and Mack (1998) suggest that when these figures are adjusted for estimates of actual age rather than age at diagnosis, the proportion of cases in the 50 and over population is closer to 15%.

As seen in Table 1, the number and proportion of AIDS cases decline in the older age groups, with less than 2% of AIDS cases being diagnosed in persons age 65 and over. One important distinction between age groups is associated with gender. While cases of AIDS in older adults decline overall, this pattern changes among older women. More women age 65 and over have been diagnosed with AIDS than those ages 60-64. Older adults in general and older adults living with HIV/ AIDS, specifically, are far from a homogeneous population. The diversity seen in age at diagnosis may also reflect differences in history, values, willingness to disclose HIV status, available social support, and help-seeking behaviors. Future demographic trends are particularly important to consider. As seen in Table 1, over 80,000 cases of AIDS have been diagnosed in individuals ages 45-49 and another 114,500 cases in those ages 40-44. With increased life expectancy from Highly Active Antiretroviral Therapies (HAART), large numbers of middle-aged individuals will be aging with HIV/AIDS in the coming years.

EPIDEMIOLOGY

While tainted blood products constituted a major source of HIV infection in the early years of the pandemic, particularly for older adults, blood products in the United States have been carefully screened since 1985, making this mode of transmission negligible (Nichols et al., 2002). Generally, older adults are exposed to HIV through the same methods as younger people including: men having sex with men, injection drug use, and heterosexual contact (CDC, 1998). There are, however, some important differences in HIV exposure for older persons as seen in Table 2. Notably, those over age 50 are slightly less likely to be exposed to HIV through men having sex with men or injection drug use, but have an increased likelihood of exposure risk through heterosexual contact, blood products or having an unknown or unidentified risk (CDC, 1998; Inungu, Mokotoff, & Kent, 2001). The decreased knowl-

TABLE 1. AIDS Cases by Sex, Age at Diagnosis, and Race/Ethnicity, Reported Through December 2001, United States

Male Age at diagnosis (years)	White, not Hispanic		Black, not Hispanic		Hispanic		Asian/Pacific Islander		American Indian/ Alaska Native		Total[1]	
	No.	%	No.	%	No.	%	No.	%	No.	%	No.	%
Under 5	535	(0)	2,165	(1)	783	(1)	17	(0)	12	(1)	3,515	(1)
5-12	346	(0)	498	(0)	284	(0)	10	(0)	6	(0)	1,146	(0)
13-19	916	(0)	1,020	(0)	570	(0)	26	(0)	23	(1)	2,555	(0)
20-24	7,938	(3)	7,590	(3)	4,520	(4)	181	(3)	84	(4)	20,337	(3)
25-29	38,967	(12)	26,595	(12)	17,138	(14)	675	(13)	351	(17)	83,794	(12)
30-34	71,345	(23)	46,088	(20)	28,377	(23)	1,161	(22)	536	(26)	147,600	(22)
35-39	71,995	(23)	51,302	(22)	27,047	(22)	1,169	(22)	473	(23)	152,124	(23)
40-44	52,653	(17)	41,395	(18)	19,215	(16)	927	(17)	303	(15)	114,585	(17)
45-49	32,116	(10)	24,839	(11)	10,937	(9)	558	(10)	134	(7)	68,635	(10)
50-54	17,498	(6)	12,959	(6)	5,861	(5)	301	(6)	63	(3)	36,718	(5)
55-59	9,337	(3)	6,987	(3)	3,242	(3)	177	(3)	37	(2)	19,801	(3)
60-64	5,139	(2)	3,819	(2)	1,769	(1)	76	(1)	18	(1)	10,829	(2)
65 or older	4,249	(1)	3,242	(1)	1,455	(1)	76	(1)	17	(1)	9,048	(1)
Male subtotal	313,034	(100)	228,499	(100)	121,198	(100)	5,354	(100)	2,057	(100)	670,687	(100)

Female Age at diagnosis (years)												
Under 5	502	(2)	2,153	(3)	770	(3)	17	(2)	13	(3)	3,460	(2)
5-12	196	(1)	521	(1)	223	(1)	10	(1)	0	(0)	953	(1)
13-19	295	(1)	1,250	(1)	316	(1)	8	(1)	4	(1)	1,873	(1)
20-24	1,774	(6)	4,844	(6)	1,625	(6)	46	(6)	36	(8)	8,328	(6)
25-29	4,831	(16)	11,876	(14)	4,364	(15)	116	(14)	69	(14)	21,266	(15)
30-34	6,818	(22)	18,055	(21)	6,418	(22)	146	(18)	105	(22)	31,564	(22)
35-39	6,244	(20)	18,351	(22)	5,878	(21)	142	(18)	95	(20)	30,733	(21)
40-44	4,199	(14)	13,221	(16)	3,950	(14)	121	(15)	61	(13)	21,560	(15)
45-49	2,307	(7)	6,922	(8)	2,249	(8)	74	(9)	48	(10)	11,607	(8)
50-54	1,309	(4)	3,447	(4)	1,245	(4)	37	(5)	22	(5)	6,062	(4)
55-59	816	(3)	1,865	(2)	750	(3)	29	(4)	18	(4)	3,479	(2)
60-64	519	(2)	1,103	(1)	411	(1)	29	(4)	5	(1)	2,069	(1)
65 or older	1,044	(3)	1,073	(1)	355	(1)	28	(3)	4	(1)	2,507	(2)
Female subtotal	30,854	(100)	84,681	(100)	28,554	(100)	803	(100)	480	(100)	145,461	(100)
Total[2]	343,889		313,180		149,752		6,157		2,537		816,149	

[1]Includes 545 males and 89 females whose race/ethnicity is unknown.
[2]Includes 1 person whose sex is unknown.
Source: Centers for Disease Control and Prevention, HIV/AIDS Surveillance Report, Year-end edition,13(2), Table 7.
Retrieved from: http://www.cdc.gov/hiv/stats/hasr1302/table7.htm

TABLE 2. AIDS Cases in the U.S., by Age Group and Exposure Category in 1996

HIV exposure category	≥ 50 years n = 7,459	13-49 years n = 61,014
Men who have sex with men	35.9%	40.4%
Injection drug use (IDU)	19.2%	25.6%
MSM and IDU	2.2%	4.6%
Heterosexual contact	14.5%	12.7%
Blood products	2.4%	1.1%
No risk reported	25.8%	15.6%

Source: Centers for Disease Control and Prevention, MMWR,1998, 47(2), 21-26.

edge of HIV transmission and limited perceptions of HIV risk among older persons may alter their ability to make informed decisions about risky sexual behavior (Nichols et al., 2002). This point is underscored by a study by El-Sadr and Gettler (1995) who examined 257 hospital patients, age 60 and over, all of whom had no previous history of HIV disease. They found 13 of those older individuals to be infected with HIV, the majority of which were women.

In addition to HIV exposure, other epidemiological issues make HIV disease different for older adults. Physiologically, older adults experience a natural senescence to their immune system that may be associated with more rapid disease progression. Specific to older women, normal aging related changes place postmenopausal women at greater risk as estrogen loss results in thinning of the vaginal mucosa, leaving them more susceptible to tears of the vaginal walls during sexual activity (Linsk, 2000; Szirony, 1999; Zelenetz & Epstein, 1998).

Once infected, epidemiological studies suggest that older adults experience a variety of complicating factors with regard to treatment and outcomes as compared to their younger counterparts. The weakened immune system mentioned previously has been suggested as a factor associated with more rapid disease progression found among older persons. Numerous studies have found shorter survival times among older persons (Ferro & Salit, 1992; Inungu, Mokotoff, & Kent, 2001), in addition to higher rates of mortality (CDC, 1998; Emlet & Farkas, 2002; Ferro & Salit, 1992).

Another important epidemiological aspect of HIV among older adults is the issue of comorbidity. The physical well-being of older persons may be impacted not only by HIV, but also by age-related diseases such as arthritis, non-HIV related respiratory or cardiac disease, or other disease processes. Skeist and Keiser (1997) found persons age 55 and over to have significantly higher rates of concurrent non-HIV related health conditions than their younger counterparts. The complication of comorbity means that older persons living with HIV disease are medically diverse and can range from being HIV+ with few symptoms to having a complex interplay of serious HIV related symptoms coupled with age related diseases. As a provider of HIV services, the first author was surprised to learn from some older clients that they were more concerned about age related chronic conditions, such as cardiac disease or diabetes, than about the management of their HIV disease.

Recent research regarding the use and efficacy of antiretroviral medications (including HAART) among older adults is encouraging. Recent research has suggested that older adults are prescribed antiretroviral therapy at equal proportions to their younger counterparts (Emlet & Berghuis, 2002; Wellons et al., 2002), and that those therapies are equally as effective (Wellons et al., 2002). In fact, Wellons and colleagues found older adults to be more compliant with HIV medication regimes than their younger counterparts. One complicating factor, however, is the increased likelihood of contraindications or drug-drug interactions between medications prescribed for HIV/AIDS and other medical conditions.

GENDER

Throughout the epidemic, men have been disproportionately affected by HIV/AIDS. This pattern holds true for adults age 50 and over. As shown in Table 1, approximately 84% of all cases of AIDS in persons 50 years and older are diagnosed in men. Older men, thus, represent a population in need of prevention and education efforts in addition to care and treatment. Because of the dominant impact on men, however, older women living with HIV/AIDS have historically been marginalized and overlooked. Little research has been conducted that examines older women relative to their risk for contracting HIV or their experiences of living with the disease (Zablotsky, 1998). Assumptions that older women are not infected with, nor impacted by, HIV/AIDS continue to exist. Contrary to these assumptions, women age 50 and over have consistently comprised approximately 9% of all cases of AIDS diagnosed in adolescent and adult females since 1993 (Zablotsky, 1998). We must recognize that women of all ages, including older women, represent a specific vulnerable population with their own needs for prevention and education. It is critical that we understand the ideologies that place older women at risk, as well as these specific care and treatment needs.

With regard to prevention and education, older women are more likely than their younger counterparts to state they know little or nothing about HIV (Zablotsky, 1998). Older women, who are no longer concerned about pregnancy, may not see a need for condom use. Yet Binson, Pollack, and Catania (1997) suggest that as many as 4.5 million women 40 or older engage in behaviors that place them at risk for HIV. Nichols and colleagues (2002) state that prevention efforts must not only include the basics of HIV/AIDS for older women, but should discuss how they can protect themselves and negotiate with sexual partners the practice of safe sex. These prevention efforts must also cover issues of power and control, the risks of drug and alcohol use, and the risk of injection drug use (Nichols et al., 2002).

Social workers and other health care providers must recognize that older women, once infected, face differences in socio-demographic characteristics that can heighten their vulnerability. For example, in a study by Schable, Chu, and Diaz (1996), women over 50 with HIV/AIDS were more likely to be widowed, separated, or divorced; and to live alone and to have less than 12 years of schooling than their younger counterparts. They were more likely to report being exposed to HIV through sex with a man whose risk of exposure was unknown and were less likely to use condoms and more likely to be tested for HIV while in the hospital (with HIV related symptoms).

Older women have been found to have different support needs than their younger, HIV-infected counterparts. Emlet, Tangenberg, and Siverson (2002) reported on participants in a support group designed specifically for older women and found they could not relate to the issues addressed in (younger) women's HIV support groups. In those groups, topics often focused on pregnancy, vertical transmission, parenting, and child care. As one woman in her mid 50s put it, "It's about time that there's a group just for older women because we have different issues, like menopause, body changes and relating to our adult children. I kind of feel left out sitting in a group hearing people talk about what their babies are doing" (p. 239).

If the needs of older, HIV-infected and at-risk women are to be met, we must recognize that older women continue to be sexually active. We must acknowledge the historical elements of poverty, racism, sexism–and more recently HIV-stigma that will continue to impact their lives. Tangenberg (2002) suggests the need for greater recognition of older women's sexuality by health and social service providers, increased HIV education for older adults, and further research on the physical, psychological and social needs of older, HIV-positive women. Media and marketing campaigns can raise awareness of HIV in older women, reinforce the needs for educational programs, and foster respect for older adults as a group (HIV Wisdom for Older Women, n.d.)

RACE/ETHNICITY

HIV/AIDS in the United States has heavily impacted people of color. In particular, African Americans and Hispanics have been disproportionately affected in recent years. As seen in Figure 1, the consistent rise in cases of AIDS among African Americans surpassed those in the non-Hispanic White population in approximately 1995. The proportion of newly reported cases among non-Hispanic whites has continually decreased while increasing in African Americans and Hispanics (CDC, 2000).

The disproportionate number of cases of AIDS and HIV infection among people of color across ages appears to hold true for those 50 and over. In examining Table 1, we can see that the majority of AIDS cases (65%) in those diagnosed at age 50 or over were among people of color, primarily African Americans and non-White Hispanics. Older women of color are particularly impacted. While 52.6% of AIDS cases among men in this age group are in people of color, the proportion among older women is 73.9%. In fact, among women ages 65 and over, more African American women have received an AIDS diagnosis than their White counterparts.

According to Brown and Sankar (1998), socio-demographic circumstances differ among elders of color, and these differences may influence how HIV/AIDS is experienced among older adults in ethnic minority communities. These differences may influence numerous issues including awareness and knowledge of HIV, sexual practices and

FIGURE 1. Proportion of AIDS Cases, by Race/Ethnicity and Year of Report, 1985-2000, United States

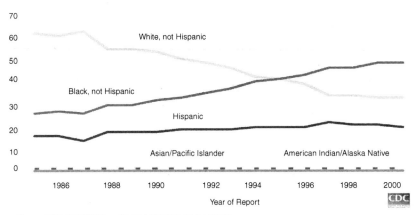

Source: CDC HIV/AIDS Surveillance L178 Slide Series (2000)

preventive behaviors, social support, access to health care, as well as service use (Brown & Sankar, 1998).

Older adults from ethnic minority communities have been found to possess lower levels of knowledge about HIV/AIDS as compared to their White counterparts of the same age (LeBlanc, 1993). Additionally, stigma associated with HIV among people of color may be a significant barrier to prevention, education and testing (Nichols et al., 2002). HIV prevention and education programs aimed specifically at older adults are rare. One example is the Senior HIV Intervention Project (SHIP) in Florida. SHIP trains older peer educators to present educational and safer sex seminars at retirement communities (University of California, San Francisco, 1997). Another HIV prevention program, the Senior HIV Prevention and Education (SHAPE), was discontinued as of December, 2002 (University of South Florida, n.d.). Prevention and education messages may not be presented in ways that are culturally sensitive or may not be presented in a fashion that older adults accept as relevant to themselves. A recent videotape, however, entitled *HIV/AIDS and Older Americans,* produced by the National Minority AIDS Council (2001), is a good example of age-sensitive messages regarding prevention and education from a multicultural perspective.

Once infected with HIV, elders of color face a variety of issues that may exacerbate support, care, and treatment. It is well-documented that elders of color experience greater morbidity and mortality due to chronic health conditions such as diabetes, hypertension and cardiovascular disease than whites (Hooyman & Kiyak, 2002). These comorbid health conditions may serve to increase functional disability and complicate their treatment and prognosis. The increased incidence of comorbidity seen among older adults in general (Skeist & Keiser, 1997) may be more pronounced among African American and Hispanic elders.

It has been well-documented that older adults in minority communities value and receive considerable informal social support from a variety of sources (Hooyman & Kiyak, 2002). Family and friends often provide both instrumental and emotional support. For many older persons, particularly African Americans, the church can be an important source of support in times of need (Hooyman & Kiyak, 2002). These assumptions, however, may not hold true with regard to older adults diagnosed with HIV/AIDS. For example, Mays and Cochran (1988) suggest that older African Americans with HIV/AIDS may face rejection from family members, friends, and religious congregations because of the socially stigmatizing behaviors typically associated with HIV disease.

This supports recent findings from Emlet (2002) who notes that in a sample of 34 adults with HIV/AIDS over the age of 50, both Hispanic and African Americans received substantially less social support from friends, neighbors, and family than their White counterparts.

While older adults from communities of color may face stigmatization and marginalization from informal social support networks, they also face barriers and challenges related to formal care and treatment. Hooyman and Kiyak (2002) suggest that cultural, economic, and structural barriers influence the use of and access to services by older adults of color. For example, the perceived stigma of using services, the fear of health care providers due to historical acts of racism, real and perceived discrimination, the lack of knowledge of services, and geographical barriers may all serve to create barriers to care. Considering these barriers exist for the population of elders of color, in general, the introduction of a stigmatizing condition such as HIV/AIDS may further serve to limit and isolate them from formal service use.

SEXUAL ORIENTATION

Older adults, like their younger counterparts, vary in sexual orientation. Although sexual orientation is often used as a proxy for HIV risk, it has influences, particularly for older adults, beyond its relevance to HIV risk. As HIV is a disease that is often sexually transmitted, older adults, service providers, and society must confront ageist views of older persons being either asexual or exclusively heterosexual. Older adults face different and specific challenges regarding HIV and AIDS as compared to their younger counterparts regardless of sexual orientation. Diversity in sexual orientation must also be seen in the context of history, cohort, and belief systems.

Older adults may have decreased sexual communication skills as compared to their younger counterparts. These differences may be the result of cohort effects that dictate what is considered "proper behavior" (University of California, San Francisco, 2000). They may be reluctant to disclose behaviors they view as being socially unacceptable and may lack negotiation skills that promote safe sex. Older women, for example, grew up prior to the sexual revolution of the 1960s and 70s and were socialized to defer to male partners. As Genke (2000) points out, many of these women are now widowed or divorced and dating again after many years. However, HIV/AIDS did not exist during their last dating experiences, thus diminishing their HIV awareness and prevention strategies. Many older adults who are in long-term monogamous relationships assume their partners to be completely faithful (University of California, San Francisco, 2000). This assumption may not always be accurate and could place both partners at risk.

Older gay and bisexual men also face unique challenges that are associated with age. Gay men age 50 and over have lived half or more of their lives before the Stonewall Rebellion1 of 1969 (Grossman, 1995). Many of these men have felt a need to hide their sexual identities throughout their lives in order to protect themselves from stigma and discrimination (Szirony, 1999; Wooten-Bielski, 1999). Morrow (2001) reminds us that older sexual minorities came of age when gay-related hate and violence was more pervasive than today, and when heterosexism and homophobia remained unchallenged (Grossman, D'Augelli, & O'Connell, 2001). According to Genke (2000), many gay men of this generation "took refuge in heterosexual marriages to shield themselves from the overwhelming fear and shame of familial disapproval and societal retribution" (p. 199). Findings from Kooperman (1993) suggest that older gay men often refuse to reach out to HIV/ AIDS education and service organizations.

Social work practitioners and educators need to be aware of their own biases and ageist beliefs related to sexuality, aging, and sexual orientation. Anderson (1998) suggests the importance of ascertaining the knowledge base of clients about HIV without assumption. "To assume that the older gay man is well-informed because of his ties to the gay and lesbian community would be a mistake" (p. 445). He reminds us that the biggest barrier to success in working with this population may be our (and our colleagues) unwillingness to overcome ageism. It is the responsibility of social workers, says Anderson, to create an environment that will encourage older persons to "share in the work of surviving HIV/AIDS" (p. 448).

PSYCHOSOCIAL ISSUES

Older adults with HIV/AIDS experience many of the same psychosocial issues as their younger counterparts, such as feeling stigmatized, marginalized, and afraid (Linsk, 2000). They may fear disclosing their diagnosis, and confront strained relationships with family and friends (Zelenetz & Epstein, 1998). They can experience lack of support from the community, dwindling financial resources, and diminished quality of life (Szirony, 1999). At the same time, older adults may also experience the intersection of ageism and HIV phobia, as well as a combination of issues and problems faced by both older adults and persons living with HIV/AIDS. These issues can be categorized as intrapersonal, interpersonal, and related to the broader service delivery system.

While many older adults living with HIV/AIDS have adjusted well to their illness, Heckman and colleagues (2002) found a "sizable minority of HIV-infected older adults" with psychological symptomatology (p. 126). In a study of 113 individuals age 45 or older with HIV or AIDS, Kalichman and colleagues (2000) found 27% reported having thought of suicide in the past week. Parallel findings come from a recent study by Heckman, Kochman, and Sikkema (in press) who found that approximately one-quarter of adults age 50 and over with HIV/AIDS reported elevated levels of depression.

Researchers have found an association between psychiatric symptomology and issues of disclosure and social support. Both studies mentioned above found an association between the symptoms being studied and lower levels of social support. As several studies have found that older persons are more likely to live alone than their younger counterparts (Crystal & Sambamoorthi, 1998; Emlet & Berghuis, in press; Emlet & Farkas, 2002), it is important to recognize that decreased social support can be a complicating and serious issue. Recently, Nokes and colleagues (2000) found older adults with HIV disease less likely than younger adults to disclose their HIV status. Although not disclosing HIV status may act as a protective mechanism against stigma, it can also serve to exacerbate social isolation–a topic particularly relevant to this population.

Older adults living with HIV disease must also face prejudice and discrimination of an ageist society as a whole. As Fowler (1999) describes, "in a society that does not respect or value the aging population, older HIV-infected people may confront social and professional bias regarding allocation of health care services and resources available to the AIDS community" (p. 4). Older adults can be caught between aging and HIV services, wherein their HIV issues may not be addressed by aging programs, while AIDS support services are typically geared to a younger population (Genke, 2000). Heckman and colleagues (in press) found decreased social support to be associated with higher barriers to health care and social services. Older adults living with HIV may be the unwitting victims of multiple programs working at cross-purposes, and lack the knowledge of where to turn for help.

CAREGIVING AND AFFECTED OLDER ADULTS

Older adults infected with the HIV virus are slowly becoming recognized as a population of elders needing care, resources and attention. Still, a growing number of older adults are what Poindexter (2001) refers to as *HIV-affected*. HIV-affected "refers to those family members who have responsibilities of caregiving for an adult or child who has HIV disease" (p. 525). Mullan (1998) suggests that age is particularly relevant to caregiving and HIV, as: (1) younger infected individuals and their caregivers are aging; (2) older people contract AIDS; and (3) older people become informal caregivers to those with HIV/AIDS. Estimates suggest as many as one-third of persons living with AIDS are dependent upon older relatives (often parents) for financial, emotional, and physical support (Allers, 1990).

Older, HIV-affected caregivers face numerous challenges and rewards for accepting their caregiving role. The caregivers own health-related and aging issues, unexpected role change, as well as stigma and disclosure, are all examples of issues than can present as problems and barriers for older caregivers. Many caregivers for persons living with HIV/AIDS are not only older, but also women of color. In these instances, the compounding effects of vulnerability and marginalization from racism, sexism, and ageism must be recognized. Additionally, however, recent research serves to remind us that taking on these caregiving roles can be a personally rewarding and even a transformative experience.

Older HIV-affected caregivers must contend with their own aging and concomitant health problems. Older caregiving grandparents often report poorer health than their non-caregiving counterparts (Joslin & Harrison, 2002) and have a higher incidence of depression (Fuller-Thomson & Minkler, 2000). In their study of 20 caregivers living in New Jersey, Joslin and Harrison (2002) reported that over half of the respondents described their health as *fair* or *poor*. These figures contrast with those nationally where 72% of adults age 65 and over rate their health as *good* or *excellent* (Federal Interagency Forum on Aging-Related Statistics, 2000). HIV caregivers also report numerous somatic symptoms including chronic fatigue, physical exhaustion, and backaches. The Joslin study found that over half of the caregivers in their sample also rated their emotional health as *fair* or *poor*. As these data suggest, HIV-affected caregivers are individuals vulnerable to physical and emotional distress.

Accepting the role as caregiver for a loved one with HIV/AIDS may initiate changes in expected or anticipated life roles. Some parent caregivers may need to confront lifestyle and behavioral aspects of their adult child's life that were heretofore ignored. For example, parents may simultaneously learn of a child's drug use or homosexuality while, at the some time, learning of their HIV or AIDS diagnosis (Levine-Perkell, 1996). Accepting the role of caregiver may require one to reassess career direction, retirement, social relationships, and the issue of "out of time" role change (Mullan, 1998). The acceptance of such change is not limited to spouses or parents of an individual with HIV/ AIDS but to grandparents as well.

As Joslin (2000) points out, catastrophic illness and death have always served as a reason for grandparents to accept parenting roles. She estimates that as many as 20,000 grandparents in the U.S. are raising approximately 41,000 children orphaned by AIDS. These grandchildren may or may not themselves be HIV-infected. Grandparents in this role often experience compromised health and well-being. Grandparent caregivers in Joslin's study reported an average of three chronic illnesses including cardiac disease, arthritis, hypertension, and diabetes. In fact, according to Joslin (2000), participants in this study from New Jersey reported poorer self-reported health than grandparents from California raising grandchildren in the wake of the crack cocaine epidemic.

Like those infected with HIV, affected caregivers confront issues of stigma and the potential benefits and detriments of disclosure. Fear of stigma and further marginalization may cause HIV-affected caregivers to limit their disclosure of HIV issues or not disclose at all. As Poindexter and Linsk (1999) suggest, disclosure of HIV must precede the experience of being stigmatized, yet it is the fear of being stigmatized that precedes disclosure. In their qualitative study of 19 older African American caregivers, Poindexter and Linsk found that ascribing the illness of the care receiver to another cause, i.e., cancer, was a common method of avoiding or minimizing stigma. In fact, none of the four caregivers in this study who were grandparents disclosed the HIV status to their infected minor grandchildren "in an effort to protect the children from feeling stigmatized" (p. 53). The fear of potential stigma may also result in the elimination of potential sources of care and support for the caregiver. Poindexter and Linsk found 11 of the participants in their study who attended church had not disclosed the issue of HIV to anyone in the church–including the pastor. As these researchers put it, "it is a tragedy that these caregivers and their HIV-positive loved ones often live in terror of disclosure and, thus, do not gain access to informal and formal support because of this fear" (pp. 57-58).

Despite the fact that many caregivers of persons with HIV or their survivors face obstacles of stigma, disclosure and physical as well as mental health problems, caregiving is not without its rewards. In a qualitative study of seven HIV-affected older caregivers, Poindexter (2001) noted that these women gained a variety of personal and societal benefits from their experience. She notes particularly the development of a strong reciprocal relationship with the HIV-positive care recipient. It was this relationship that sustained the caregivers and helped them get through their challenges. Another positive result in her study was the commitment to social justice by the caregivers. They developed "impassioned belief in the right of adults and children with HIV to participate fully in society and not be neglected" (p. 530). Some caregivers have called this experience transformative.

Although early in the epidemic, much of the literature and research on HIV caregivers focused on gay men and their infected partners, caregivers have become much more diverse in the past three decades. We recognize that HIV-affected caregivers vary in relationship to the care recipient, and represent diversity in gender, ethnicity, and age. Types of coping strategies, informal support networks, and willingness to seek formal services may depend upon history, knowledge, and trust (or lack of) in the health and social service system.

CONCLUSIONS

The purpose of this paper was to help enlighten social workers, students, and educators regarding the heterogeneous makeup of older persons infected with and affected by HIV/AIDS. As we have seen from this brief review, older persons experience physiological, psychological and historical differences as compared to their younger counterparts. Older adults living with HIV/AIDS vary in age, gender, ethnicity, sexual orientation, and exposure to HIV. Ageist and sexist stereotypes will need to be confronted by all as we move more fully into the 21st century and see a continued increase in the numbers of older persons becoming infected and living with HIV/AIDS. Additionally, the confounding intersection of racism, ageism, sexism, homophobia and HIV-stigma will continue to create tremendous barriers for these older adults. The social work profession must recognize this growing population of vulnerable elders as individuals with special needs requiring a sensitive and knowledgeable approach to care.

Social workers must also recognize the diverse population that makes up HIV-affected caregivers. Because many of these caregivers are older women of color, they have likely faced discrimination and prejudice throughout their lives. For older persons both infected with and affected by HIV, better communication and coordination between health and social service systems will need to be forged. Professionals providing services designed for persons living with HIV will need to better understand the needs of their older consumers, while the *aging network* will need to recognize the differences and special needs of an emerging and diverse population of vulnerable older adults.

REFERENCES

Allers, C. T. (1990). AIDS and the older adult. *The Gerontologist, 30*, 405-407.

Anderson, G. (1998). Providing services to elderly people with HIV. In D. M. Aronstein & B. J. Thompson (Eds.), *HIV and social work: A practitioner's guide* (pp. 443-450). New York: The Harrington Park Press.

Binson, D., Pollack, L., & Catania, J. A. (1997). AIDS-related risk behaviors and safe sex practices of women in midlife and older in the United States: 1990 to 1992. *Health Care for Women International, 18*(4), 343-354.

Brown, D. R., & Sankar, A. (1998). HIV/AIDS and aging minority populations. *Research on Aging, 20*, 865-884.

Centers for Disease Control and Prevention (1998). AIDS among persons aged ≥ 50 years–United States, 1991-1996. *Morbidity and Mortality Weekly Report, 47*(2), 21-27.

Centers for Disease Control and Prevention (2000). *HIV/AIDS Surveillance–General Epidemiology, L178 slide series (through 2000), slide #8.* Retrieved December 26, 2002 from the World Wide Web: *http://www.cdc.gov/hiv/graphics/surveill.htm.*

Centers for Disease Control and Prevention (CDC) (2002). *HIV/AIDS Surveillance Report, year end edition, 13*(2), 1-41.

Crystal, S., & Sambamoorthi, U. (1998). Health care needs and service delivery for older persons with HIV/AIDS: Issues and research challenges. *Research on Aging, 20*, 739-759.

El-Sadr, W., & Gettler, J. (1995). Unrecognized human immunodeficiency virus infection in the elderly. *Archives of Internal Medicine, 155*, 184-186.

Emlet, C. A. (1997). HIV/AIDS in the elderly: A hidden population. *Home Care Provider, 2*, 69-75.

Emlet, C. A. (2002, November). Older adults living with HIV/AIDS: An emerging vulnerable population. Paper presented as part of the symposium *Emergent issues in contexts of care for vulnerable populations of elders.* The 55th Annual Scientific Meeting of the Gerontological Society of America. Boston, MA.

Emlet, C. A., & Berghuis, J. P. (2002). Service priorities, use and needs: Views of older and younger consumers living with HIV/AIDS. *Journal of Mental Health and Aging,* *8*(4), 307-318.

Emlet, C. A., & Farkas, K. J. (2002). Correlates of service utilization among midlife and older adults with HIV/AIDS: The role of age in the equation. *Journal of Aging and Health, 14,* 315-335.

Emlet, C. A., Tangenberg, K., & Siverson, C. (2002). A feminist approach to practice in working with mid-life and older women with HIV/AIDS. *Affilia: Journal of Women and Social Work, 17,* 229-251.

Federal Interagency Forum on Aging Related Statistics (2000). *Older Americans 2000: Key indicators of well-being.* Washington, DC: Author.

Ferro, S., & Salit, I. E. (1992). HIV infection in patients over 55 years of age. *Journal of Acquired Immune Deficiency Syndrome, 5,* 348-355.

Fowler, J. P. (1999). HIV in people over 50. *Focus: A Guide to AIDS Research and Counseling, 14*(9), 1-4.

Fuller-Thomson, E., & Minkler, M. (2000). The mental and physical health of grandmothers who are raising their grandchildren. *Journal of Mental Health and Aging,* *6*(4), 311-323.

Genke, J. (2000). HIV/AIDS and older adults: The invisible ten percent. *Care Management Journals, 2*(3), 196-205.

Grossman, A. H. (1995). At risk, infected, and invisible: Older gay men and HIV/AIDS. *Journal of the Association of Nurses in AIDS Care, 6*(6), 13-19.

Grossman, A. H., D'Augelli, A. R., & O'Connell, T. S. (2001). Being lesbian, gay, bisexual and 60 or older in North America. *Journal of Gay and Lesbian Social Services, 13*(4), 23-40.

Heckman, T. G., Heckman, B. D., Kochman, A., Sikkema, K. J., Suhr, J., & Goodkin, K. (2002). Psychological symptoms among persons 50 years of age and older living with HIV disease. *Aging and Mental Health, 6*(2), 121-128.

Heckman, T. G., Kochman, A., & Sikkema, K. J. (in press). Depressive symptoms in older adults living with HIV disease: Application of the chronic illness quality of life model. *Journal of Mental Health and Aging, 8*(4).

HIV Wisdom for Older Women (n.d.). *Things you should know about HIV and older women.* Retrieved April 17, 2003 from the world wide web: *http://www.hivwisdom. org/facts.html.*

Hooyman, N. R., & Kiyak, H. A. (2002). *Social gerontology: A multidisciplinary perspective* (6th edition). Boston: Allyn and Bacon.

Inungu, J. N., Mokotoff, E. D., & Kent, J. B. (2001). Characteristics of HIV infection in patients fifty years or older in Michigan. *AIDS Patient Care and STDs, 15,* 567-573.

Joslin, D. (2000). Grandparents raising children orphaned and affected by HIV/AIDS. In C. Cox (Ed.), *To grandmother's house we go and stay: Perspectives on custodial grandparents* (pp. 167-183). New York: Springer.

Joslin, D., & Harrison, R. (2002). Physical health and emotional well-being. In D. Joslin (Ed.), *Invisible caregivers: Older adults raising children in the wake of HIV/AIDS* (pp. 90-112). New York: Columbia University Press.

Kalichman, S. C., Heckman, T., Kochman, A., Sikkema, K., & Bergholte, J. (2000). Depression and thoughts of suicide among middle-aged and older persons living with HIV-AIDS. *Psychiatric Services, 51*(7), 903-907.

Kooperman, L. (1993, March). *AIDS and the elderly.* Paper presented at the 39th Annual Meeting of the American Society on Aging. Chicago.

LeBlanc, A. J. (1993). Examining HIV-related knowledge among adults in the US. *Journal of Health and Social Behavior, 34,* 23-36.

Levine-Perkell, J. (1996). Caregiving Issues. In K. Nokes (Ed.), *HIV/AIDS and the older adult* (pp. 115-128). Bristol, PA: Taylor and Francis.

Linsk, N. L. (2000). HIV among older adults: Age-specific issues in prevention and treatment. *The AIDS Reader, 10*(7), 430-440.

Mays, V. M., & Cochran, S. D. (1988). Issues in the perception of AIDS risk and risk reduction activities by Black and Hispanic women. *American Psychology, 43,* 949-957.

Morrow, D. F. (2001). Older gays and lesbians: Surviving a generation of hate and violence. *Journal of Gay and Lesbian Social Services, 13*(1/2), 151-169.

Mullan, J. T. (1998). Aging and informal caregiving to people with HIV/AIDS. *Research on Aging, 20,* 712-738.

National Minority AIDS Council (Producer) (2001). *HIV/AIDS and older Americans* [Video recording]. (Available from the National Minority AIDS Council, 1931 13th Street, N.W. Washington, DC, 20009)

Nichols, J. E., Speer, D. C., Watson, B. J., Watson, M. R., Vergon, T. L., Valee, C. M., & Meah, J. M. (2002*). Aging with HIV: Psychological, social and health issues.* San Diego: Academic Press.

Nokes, K. M., Holzemer, W. L., Corless, I. B., Bakken, S., Brown, M.-A., Powell-Cope, G. M., Inouye, J., & Turner, J. (2000). Health-related quality of life in persons younger and older than 50 who are living with HIV/AIDS. *Research on Aging, 22,* 290-310.

Ory, M. G., & Mack, K. A. (1998). Middle-aged and older people with AIDS. *Research on Aging, 20,* 653-664.

Poindexter, C. C. (2001). "I'm still blessed": The assets and needs of HIV-affected caregivers over 50. *Families in Society, 82*(5), 525-536.

Poindexter, C. C., & Linsk, N. L. (1999). HIV-related stigma in a sample of HIV-affected older female African American caregivers. *Social Work, 44,* 46-61.

Riley, M. W. (1989). AIDS and older people: The overlooked segment of the population. In M. W. Riley, M. G. Ory, & D. Zablotsky (Eds.), *AIDS in an aging society: What we need to know* (pp. 3-26). New York: Springer.

Schable, B., Chu, S., & Diaz, T. (1996). Characteristics of women 50 years of age and older with heterosexually acquired AIDS. *American Journal of Public Health, 86,* 1616-1618.

Skeist, D. J., & Keiser, P. (1997). Human immunodeficiency virus infection in patients older than 50 years. *Archives of Family Medicine, 6*(3), 289-294.

Szirony, T. A. (1999). Infection with HIV in the elderly population. *Journal of Gerontological Nursing, 25*(10), 25-31.

Tangenberg, K. M. (2002). Mental health dimensions of HIV/AIDS in women over 50. *Journal of Mental Health and Aging, 8*(4), pp. 281-294.

University of California-San Francisco (2000). HIV and older adults. *HIV Counselor Perspectives*, 9(5), 1-7.

University of California-San Francisco (1997). *What are the prevention needs of adults over 50?* Center for AIDS Prevention Studies, University of California-San Francisco. Fact Sheet # 29E.

University of South Florida. (n.d.). *Department of Aging and Mental Health, SHAPE Project* Update. Retrieved April 17, 2003 from the world wide web: *http://amhserver. fmhi.usf.edu/shape/index.html.*

Wellons, M. F., Sanders, L., Edwards, L. J., Bartlett, J. A., Heald, A. E., & Schmader, K. E. (2002). HIV infection: Treatment outcomes in older and younger adults. *Journal of the American Geriatrics Society*, 50, 603-607.

Wooten-Bielski, K. (1999). HIV & AIDS in older adults. *Geriatric Nursing*, 20(5), 268-272.

Zablotsky, D. L. (1998). Overlooked, ignored and forgotten: Older women at risk for HIV infection and AIDS. *Research on Aging, 20*, 760-775.

Zelenetz, P. D., & Epstein, M. E. (1998). HIV in the elderly. *AIDS Patient Care and STD's, 12*(4), 255-262.

CAREGIVERS

Grandparents Raising Grandchildren: A Diverse Population

Nancy P. Kropf
Stacey Kolomer

SUMMARY. The number of grandparents who are raising grandchildren has risen dramatically as the result of several social trends. Within this article, diversity aspects of this population are explored including characteristics of the grandparents and grandchildren. In addition, support groups, the primary intervention for custodial grandparents, are overviewed with specific attention to models that have relevance for subpopulations of care providers. Finally, child welfare and kinship care policies are examined and critiqued from a diversity perspective. *[Article copies available for a fee from The Haworth Document Delivery Service: 1-800-HAWORTH. E-mail address: <docdelivery@haworthpress.com> Website: <http://www.HaworthPress.com> © 2004 by The Haworth Press, Inc. All rights reserved.]*

Nancy P. Kropf, PhD, is Professor, School of Social Work and Associate Vice President for Instruction, and Stacey Kolomer, PhD, is Assistant Professor, School of Social Work, both at University of Georgia, Athens, GA 30602.

[Haworth co-indexing entry note]: "Grandparents Raising Grandchildren: A Diverse Population." Kropf, Nancy P., and Stacey Kolomer. Co-published simultaneously in *Journal of Human Behavior in the Social Environment* (The Haworth Social Work Practice Press, an imprint of The Haworth Press, Inc.) Vol. 9, No. 4, 2004, pp. 65-83; and: *Diversity and Aging in the Social Environment* (eds: Sherry M. Cummings, and Colleen Galambos) The Haworth Social Work Practice Press, an imprint of The Haworth Press, Inc., 2004, pp. 65-83. Single or multiple copies of this article are available for a fee from The Haworth Document Delivery Service [1-800-HAWORTH. 9:00 a.m. - 5:00 p.m. (EST). E-mail address: docdelivery@haworthpress.com].

http://www.haworthpress.com/web/JHBSE
© 2004 by The Haworth Press, Inc. All rights reserved.
Digital Object Identifier: 10.1300/J137v09n04_04

KEYWORDS. Grandparents, elderly, grandchildren, race, gender

Although grandparents have historically assumed roles in caring for their grandchildren, the number of grandparents in primary caregiving roles has increased dramatically. A national probability sample of grandmothers indicates that 43% provide supportive child care for grandchildren (Baydar & Brooks-Gunn, 1998). Of particular interest, however, is the number of grandparents who have primary responsibility for raising grandchildren. Current estimates of these "custodial grandparents" indicate that about 5-6% of children live in households with grandparents, with about 10% of grandparents having responsibility to raise children (Pebley & Rudkin, 1999).

Caregiving grandparents (also called "custodial grandparents") are a diverse group of individuals. One commonality, however, is the unexpected experience that many custodial grandparents share in having child-raising responsibility again. The impact of this unexpected and/or unplanned event has different outcomes for grandparents as a result of their characteristics and life situations. This article will present an overview of the diversity that is found within the custodial grandparent population, and discuss social work practice and policy for this group.

DIVERSE CHARACTERISTICS
OF CUSTODIAL GRANDPARENTS

The experience of raising children is one that impacts various dimensions of a grandparent's life. Various outcomes appear to cut across experiences within the general population of custodial grandparents. Outcomes include a decrease in overall health and well-being of these grandparents, as raising grandchildren involves physically and emotionally demanding tasks (Bowers & Myers, 1999; Fuller-Thomson & Minkler, 2000; Jendrek, 1994; Musil, 1998; Szinovascz, DeViney, & Atkinson, 1999). Social well-being may also suffer, as less time and energy is available for social contacts and other relationships (Minkler, Roe, & Robertson-Beckley, 1994; Strawbridge, Wallhagen, Shema, & Kaplan, 1997). These consequences can create difficulty in grandparents' lives, and physical and emotional functioning.

There are caregiving aspects, however, that are more associated with certain profiles of grandparents. For the purpose of this article, aspects of diversity within this population will be explored including race/ethnicity, age, gender, and geographic location. In addition, service and policy-related issues which are relevant for custodial grandparents will be highlighted and critiqued.

Race/Ethnicity

While custodial grandparents are represented in all racial and ethnic groups, African American and Latino grandparents are disproportionately represented within this population (Caputo, 1999; Fuller-Thomson, Minkler, & Driver, 1997). For this reason, one area of research with custodial grandparents has identified aspects of care provision for grandparents by racial/ethnic groups. Studies have focused on the experience of African American and Latino grandparents, and have compared their experiences to their White counterparts.

African American grandparents. An historical review of the grandparent role in African American families demonstrates that these family members have served an important role in caring for children. One function of African American grandparents has been as "kinkeepers" within the family, providing support during times of economic and social stresses such as slavery, or migration to other geographic areas for greater labor force opportunities (Burton & Dilworth-Anderson, 1991; Hunter & Taylor, 1998). Compared to White grandparents, African Americans are "less likely than Whites to embrace norms of noninterference" with higher probability that they will be involved in supporting and providing resources to younger generations within their families (Pruchno, 1999, p. 211). In kinship care arrangements, family boundaries may be quite fluid with the grandparents maintaining an informal custodial arrangement with the grandchildren. In addition, it is not uncommon to have the children's parents enter and exit the family system with some regularity (Baird, John, & Hayslip, 2000).

As social conditions have changed, however, the context and roles within families where grandparents raise children have also shown marked differences. The most prevalent reason for African American grandparents to be in custodial caregiving roles is the drug addiction of their own child. Crack cocaine abuse, in particular, has been a major factor within these families (Minkler et al., 1994). When a son or daughter is addicted to crack, children may experience abuse, neglect or maltreatment as a result of the parent's addiction. Grandparents often have additional struggles in raising children from these backgrounds, as they may exhibit challenging behavioral manifestations as a result of associated trauma.

In addition to child-rearing challenges, other stressors have been reported by African American grandparents. These caregivers incur psychological, emotional, social and financial stress within their caregiving roles (Burton, 1992). This stress is particularly acute for many African American grandparents, especially grandmothers, who have experienced the "triple jeopardy" experience of being Black, female, and in late life. A life long experience of oppression and discrimination in social and economic roles creates a limited buffer for these caregivers when they assume a caregiving role for grandchildren.

In addition, the responsibility of raising grandchildren may attenuate the grandparent's social network which can lead to feelings of burden and depression. In addition, health problems may be exacerbated or occur as a result of child-raising demands (Minkler, Roe, & Price, 1992). While these stresses are experienced for many African American grandparents, those who are in "off time" caregiving roles (e.g., are beyond the usual time frame for parenting) are especially at risk for these stressful experiences (Burton, 1996).

Latino grandparents. Similar to African Americans, Latinos are disproportionately represented in the population of custodial grandparents. One national study on custodial grandparents estimated that Latinos comprise about 10% of relative caregivers (Chalfie, 1994). In addition to the sheer number, the ethnicities represented in this group of caregivers is diverse and include Puerto Rican, Dominican, Cuban, Mexican, Ecuadorian, Honduran, Panamanian, and Nicaraguan grandparents. Within the Latino population, there is considerable diversity in terms of cultural practices and other social factors.

Combined with the "typical stresses" of caregiving, these grandparents often struggle with language and acculturation difficulties (Burnette, 1999). Quite obvious are the problems that grandparents encounter due to language barriers, including interacting with their grandchildren's school, health providers, and other services. In addition, the cultural norms may pose barriers in help-seeking behaviors of these grandparents, especially the grandmothers. There is a Latino cultural expectation that "women should be self-sufficient and must not show vulnerability by disclosing family problems outside the home environment" (Cox, Brooks, & Valcarcel, 2000, p. 227). This attitude can add to the isolation, alienation and shame that is experienced by grandparents who are in a care provision role.

Comparisons by race/ethnicity. In order to identify unique and common experiences, research on custodial grandparents has compared caregivers by race/ethnicity. Typically, research focuses on the consequences of caregiving; that is, the impact of this role on the grandparent's social, physical, and emotional functioning. In addition, the experience of support from both informal and formal sources has also been a major theme.

Some important similarities exist in the experiences of custodial grandparents. In a study comparing African American and White grandparents, several areas of commonality were reported (Pruchno, 1999). One shared stressor was balancing work demands and child care, such as having to miss work or leave early, and being unavailable outside of school hours. Regardless of race, grandparents reported high levels of satisfaction in their role performance. Similarly, neither African American nor White married grandparents reported detrimental consequences of child care on their relationship with their spouse.

Differences have been found in the experiences of custodial grandparents by race/ethnicity, however. African American grandparents are more likely than Whites to have friends who are raising grandchildren, which may decrease the sense of isolation in this role (Pruchno, 1999). In addition, another study that examined caregiving in African American and White families reported a greater degree of caregiving burden in White families (Pruchno & McKenney, 2000). Interesting, other predictors of burden (besides race) were being in a relationship (e.g., married or partnered), raising grandchildren with problematic behaviors, being in poorer health, and having poorer relationships with the child's father. This finding suggests that both personal factors and family dynamics may play a larger role in defining the caregiving outcome for White grandparents who are raising grandchildren.

In comparisons that included Latino grandparents, this group was especially at risk for poverty and lack of resources. In one study comparing African Americans, Latinos, and White grandparents, Latinos had the highest poverty rate (33% of the sample) and the lowest educational attainment (Goodman & Silverstein, 2002). For some, the lack of a legal immigration status compounds their dire economic situation as they are ineligible to receive various forms of social supports.

Gender

As in other caregiving situations, females overwhelming assume the custodial grandparent role. In establishing a caregiving hierarchy, studies suggest that most non-parent kin caregivers are grandmothers, followed next by aunts (Burnette, 1997; Dressel & Barnhill, 1994). Studies including grandparents of both genders consistently report that females greatly outnumber men, with estimates in study samples ranging from

77% to 86% being grandmothers (Fuller-Thompson et al., 1997; Hayslip, Shore, Henderson, & Lambert, 1998; Silverstein & Vehvilainen, 1998). Clearly, this is another caregiving situation that is predominantly filled by women.

The experience of men in custodial grandparent roles has started to be explored, albeit in limited ways. In a study of 33 grandfathers who participated in two grandparent support programs in the Northeast, the experience of caring for grandchildren was compared to grandmothers who also were program participants (Kolomer & McCallion, under review). These grandfathers were either primary caregivers, or jointly caring for their grandchildren with their spouses. Results indicated that caregiving grandfathers were more likely to be White, married, working outside the home, and home owners compared to custodial grandmothers. In addition, depression scores were clinically significant for grandmothers but not for the grandfathers. Through focus group discussions conducted with these grandfathers, several caregiving stressors were reported including a loss of free time, worries about future care for the grandchildren, and having health concerns.

Grandchildren may also experience their relationship with their grandfather differently than the one with their grandmother. In research with grandchildren who were being raised by grandparents, the children reported that grandfathers played a less significant role in their lives than their grandmothers (Hayslip, Shore, & Henderson, 2000). Differences seem to be gender related, however, as female children reported the most salient relationships with grandmothers while male children reported more parity in their relationships with both grandparents. Clearly, the role and experience of grandfathers who are raising grandchildren is an area where additional research is warranted.

Age

Grandparenting is a generational, not an age-based, role within the family. Therefore, a grandparent can be a thirty-five or ninety-year-old person. In addition, custodial grandparents may actually be the children's great-grandparent, as often these two roles are aggregated within the research. The timing and transition that occur within intergenerational caregiving situations have an impact on the experience and outcome for the care providers with "off time care" creating role stress and overload (Burton, 1996). However, studies on custodial grandparenting often include age as a variable for sample description, without investigating the experience of caregiving at different life phases.

The limited research in this area suggests that older care providers experience greater difficulty in role performance. In a study of rural grandparents, older caregivers in the sample reported greater physical and mental health problems than the younger ones (Robinson, Kropf, & Myers, 2000). As Burnette (1997) states, "Grandparents who are engaged in their own age-appropriate developmental tasks may be psychologically or physically unprepared to assume this level of responsibility, particularly given the challenging circumstances of this role" (p. 494).

Geographic Location

Although the majority of research on custodial grandparents has been conducted in urban areas, grandparent caregiving is not limited to these communities. One estimate indicates that about 25% of skipped generation families live in rural areas (Fuller-Thomson et al., 1997). While rural areas and small towns are sometimes perceived as idyllic, these communities experience various social problems including poverty, limited resources, and geographic isolation.

The experience of rural grandparents has some unique aspects, when compared to custodial grandparents in more urban areas. Transition issues may be especially stressful for the grandchildren, who may be leaving more urban settings to live with grandparents in smaller communities. Behaviors, norms, and experiences of children and adolescents that are accepted in urban locations (e.g., diverse lifestyles, clothing) may be shunned in smaller locations (Myers, Kropf, & Robinson, 2002). The isolation of children from peers can make the transition especially difficult for all members of the household.

Grandparents in rural communities may also struggle with locating and accessing resources to assist them in caring for their grandchildren. In research on mental health of grandparents in rural areas, findings indicated that these grandparents had low levels of both informal and formal support (Robinson et al., 2000). School districts, which may be a source of aid in some communities, seem especially unprepared to interact with grandparents in more rural areas. In addition, other sources of support (e.g., support groups, case management programs) are unlikely to be found in rural communities.

DIVERSITY OF GRANDCHILDREN RAISED
BY THEIR GRANDPARENTS

In addition to the forms of diversity that exist within the population of custodial grandparents, grandchildren are also a heterogeneous group. The characteristics of the children include both behavior and medical issues, which are often related to the reasons that they are in the care of their grandparents. As a result, these children may present additional challenges for the grandparents within their care provision role.

Health Related Concerns

One pathway into care with grandparents is HIV/AIDS, as an increasing number of children and adolescents are being raised by grandparents because of parental illness or death. These youngsters, termed "AIDS orphans" (Michaels & Levine, 1992), have experienced social and emotional trauma through the illness (and possibly death) of their parent. In addition, they may be HIV-infected themselves which may create additional physical and emotional concerns within the family. Caring for a grandchild who is HIV+ also creates emotional stresses for the grandparents such as anticipatory grief at the prospect of losing grandchildren to this disease, and keeping this medical condition secret as a way to avoid the stigma that is still associated with HIV/AIDS (Caliandro & Hughes, 1998; Pinson-Milburn, Fabian, Schlossberg, & Pyle, 1996; Poindexter & Linsk, 1999).

The disability status of a grandchild is another situation that many grandparents face. Due to the high prevalence of addiction in the etiology of grandparent caregiving, it is not surprising that the children in these families may have medical conditions that are a result of prenatal alcohol or drug exposure. In studies of White and African American custodial grandparents who were raising grandchildren with and without disabilities, grandparents with disabled grandchildren reported greater unmet service needs and depressive symptoms (Brown & Boyce-Mathis, 2000; Force, Botsford, Pisano, & Holbert, 2000; Kolomer, McCallion, & Janicki, 2002). In addition, transfer of care issues (e.g., residential placement, quality of substitute care) are particularly stressful for older parents who remain in their caregiving role for sons or daughters with disabilities (Kelly & Kropf, 1995; Kropf, 1997). The worries and fears that exist with older parents most probably create anxiety for custodial grandparents as well.

Behavioral Challenges

In addition to health related issues, some grandparents experience the challenges of raising a child with difficult behaviors. Pinson-Milburn et al. (1996) outline the various events experienced within the lives of children and adolescents who are being raised by grandparents, and some of the emotional and behavioral consequences. One is the sense of shame that children may experience as a result of living with a grand-parent. This feeling may be evident when a grandparent attends routine functions (e.g., PTA meeting, Little League game) where there is an obvious difference between these caregivers and the parents of their peers. Children may also feel a sense of difference and isolation from peers. This feeling was demonstrated by a young girl who participated in a support program for grandchildren being raised by grandparents. During the first outing of the group, she saw another grandmother walking her grandchild to one of the program vans, and she loudly exclaimed, "Oh look, she lives with her grandmother too!" (Robinson & Kropf, 2001). This experience was a normalizing one for her, and provided a mirroring of her family life by one of her young peers.

Children also may express the feelings of abandonment and anger toward their absent parent, and may also have psychiatric or physical health conditions that are a consequence of pre- and post-natal parental drug or alcohol abuse. These conditions are difficult ones for any care provider to handle, and may be especially problematic for grandparents in mid- or late-life who have fewer physical and social resources to be able to manage them effectively.

SUPPORT GROUP INTERVENTIONS

As already described, becoming a primary caregiver to a grandchild can lead to additional stressors and strains in the life of a grandparent. Some of these strains include physical problems, financial difficulty, limited housing space, regret, bereavement, and social isolation (Emick & Hayslip, 1999; Kelley, Yorker, & Whitley, 1997; Kolomer & McCallion, under review; Silverstein & Vehvilainen, 1998). Grandparent care-givers are also at higher risk for depression and anxiety disorders than other groups (Flint & Perez-Porter, 1997; Generations United, 1999; Janicki et al., 2000; Kelley et al., 1997; Kolomer, 2000; Phillips & Bloom, 1998; Roe et al., 1996). To alleviate these psychosocial conditions, many researchers and practitioners have strongly recommended the use of support groups for grandparent caregivers (Burton, 1992; Dressel, & Barnhill, 1994; Kolomer, McCallion, & Overendyer, 2003; Minkler & Roe, 1993; Myers et al., 2002).

Peer-led support groups are one type of group that has been widely utilized by grandparent caregivers. The goals of these groups are providing mutual support, eliminating isolation, and sharing the challenges of raising grandchildren with others in similar situations. There are over 400 such groups registered with AARP's Grandparent Caregiver Information Center such as Relatives as Parents Program (RAPP), Grandparents as Parents (GAP), and Raising Our Children's Kids (ROCK) (Strom & Strom, 1993). In addition to mutual aid, many groups provide important information regarding guardianship and custody issues, child care, how to work with a child's school, and other legal matters.

Groups have also been started that target a specific grandparent caregiving population that use professionals as group leaders. Cox (2002) designed a support/education group specifically for empowering African American grandparent caregivers and then replicated the same model with Latino grandparents. This model provides grandparents with information and education, with an additional outcome of having the caregivers themselves become resource and peer educators for other custodial grandparents. The participants in the group had significant input into the design of the curriculum of the 12-week course. Following the completion of the group, several of the grandparents made presentations to other grandparent caregiver support groups thereby spreading the goal of empowerment.

McCallion and colleagues (2000) designed and implemented an intervention for grandparents caring for children with developmental disabilities. The intervention consisted of case management services and support/education groups. Participants were primarily African American or Latino, and were living in inner cities. Case management services included, but were not limited to, connecting families with health services, entitlements, summer camps, housing, and interfacing with schools. The six-to-eight-week support group meetings focused on content and information identified by the participants as critical information for their role as care providers. Content included custody issues, information about developmental disabilities and available services, relaxation techniques, understanding school systems, and working with the child's biological parent. Pre- and post-tests of the grandparent caregivers showed significant decreases in depressive symptoms, and increased locus of control (Kolomer et al., 2002).

Schools are increasingly being used as a resource for recruiting grand-parent caregivers to group interventions. Burnette (1998) targeted African American and Latino grandparents in an inner city school to participate in a psychoeducation/support group. Information about local, regional, and national resources was provided to the grandparents and discussion focused on stressors, supports, managing family conflict, parenting skills training, legal options, entitlement programs, advocacy, and community-based initiatives. Following participation in the support group, the grandparents' scores for depressive symptoms improved.

For African American and Latino grandparent families, the need for strong community supports is necessary to maintain the family unit. In society today, challenges and conditions have changed so that the informal supports that once existed are unavailable (McCallion, Janicki, & Grant-Griffin, 1997; Kolomer et al., 2003). As Cox states, "Lifelong histories of poverty, low incomes, poor health status, discrimination, and poorer physical functioning exacerbate the caregiving needs" (2002, p. 46). Program planners need to design culturally responsive programs (Chenoweth, 2000). Although all of the programs that were described were designed by researchers, the caregiving grandparents had tremendous input into the programs. Grandparent caregivers should play a larger role in the design and implementation of their own services and resources.

PUBLIC POLICY INITIATIVES

While greater numbers of grandparents are raising grandchildren, public policies have not been enacted that support the diversity of care arrangements within family systems. Policy initiatives often make assumptions about families, such as care will be permanent or biological parents are totally uninvolved with the children, that are untrue for some families. When considering grandparents of color, the value and meaning of their "family" may be inconsistent with the concept which provides the foundation for legislation. Within this section, major policy initiatives that are part of informal caregiving arrangements, and those associated with more permanent arrangements, will be highlighted and critiqued.

Informal Caregiving Arrangements

Most instances of custodial caregiving are done within an informal custody arrangement, which means that grandparents have "Physical

Custody," as opposed to "Legal Custody" of the child. Typically, the parents maintain the rights over the child which opens real possibilities that the parent(s) can reassume custody of the child at any point (Albert, 2000; Flint & Perez-Porter, 1997). This possibility is troubling to many grandparents, who live with a real fear that their grandchild may return to substandard or harmful conditions if a parent chooses. Grandparents in informal caregiving roles may also have limited access to decision-making, as in school systems or medical situations (Flint & Perez-Porter, 1997).

An option to enhance decision-making capacity is to have the grandparents pursue legal custody or legal guardianship. *Legal custody* allows the grandparent to make day-to-day decisions without having control over the child's property or financial responsibility. *Legal guardians* have decision-making capacity, but the parents' rights are still maintained (Flint & Perez-Porter, 1997). The requirement to legalize the caregiving relationship may be especially dystonic for families of color who have deep meaning systems attached to the concept of "family." Historically, African Americans have taken in grandchildren, nieces, nephews, and even orphans in times of need (Burton, 1992; Kolomer et al., 2002) which makes government interference in family matters seem inconceivable. Yet, without a formal arrangement, grandparents are limited in the ability to access the necessary resources and services for their grandchildren.

Kinship Foster Care

In the past 25 years, the Federal Government has put into place several policies, ostensibly to keep children with their families of origin or within a family which most closely resembles their own cultural heritage. However, additional sets of circumstances existed including a weakening of the foster care system which resulted from changing labor force trends of women, low recruitment of foster families, proliferation of lawsuits in child welfare, an increase in child abuse/neglect reports, and increased intensity of children who needed placement (Dubowitz, Feigelman, Harrington, Starr, & Zuravin, 1994; Ingram, 1996; Kolomer, 2000). The challenge of finding appropriate placements was further intensified by the dramatic increase in substance abuse, poverty, homelessness, and HIV infection within families who had children that needed foster care (Anderson, 1990; Burnette, 1997; McGowen & Studt, 1991). By utilizing relatives as caregivers, the demand for foster families could be alleviated.

Maintaining children in cultural communities. A trend within child welfare has been to keep children within their cultural communities. The Indian Child Welfare Act of 1978 was the first law based upon this cultural assumption. This Act was designed to maintain tribal authority over the placement of Indian children as a high percentage of Native American families were misserved by agencies that lacked an understanding of Native American culture and history (*Wabanki Legal News,* 2002). The law allowed Native American children needing placement to remain within their own community and remain connected to their culture.

Another Act, Adoption Assistance and Child Welfare Act of 1980 (Public Law 96-272) defined "permanency planning" as a goal for children at risk of or who have been removed from their parents' care (Burnette, 1997). Emphasis was placed on "a set of goal-directed activities designed to help children live in families that offer continuity of relationships with nurturing parents or caretakers and the opportunity to establish lifetime relationships" (Maluccio, Fein, & Olmstead, 1986, p. 5). This policy introduced the concept of children being placed with relatives as the placement of choice. The year before the Adoption Assistance and Child Welfare Act was enacted, the Supreme Court barred the exclusion of relatives from the Foster Care System thereby giving permission for states to use relatives as foster families (*Miller v. Youakim*) (Burnette, 1997).

In spite of policies that aimed at preserving the bonds between children and their culture and family, gaps exist in the intent and outcome of policy initiatives. For example, some states require that kinship foster homes follow the same rules and regulations as required of traditional foster homes; including have case managers for the family or required parent-training courses (Kolomer, 2000). These policies are viewed as intrusive for some families, and impact the relationships and affectional ties between members. African American families who have a long history with interfering public policy, for instance, may harbor mistrust about the intention of these policy initiatives. In addition, caregivers may face criticism by others in their community for accepting government funding for what is seen as a moral responsibility to take in family members during times of need (Crumbley & Little, 1997; Kolomer, 2000).

Time limitations in care. Other child welfare policy addresses time limits for children within foster care. The Adoption and Safe Families Act of 1997 provides guidelines to limit the time children can stay wards of the state (Albert, 2000). Within 12 to 15 months of entering the foster care system, "reasonable efforts" must be made to reunite a child with his or her biological parents. If unsuccessful, parental rights must be terminated.

While the intention to prevent foster care drift is a good one, this policy does not consider the norms of diverse racial/ethnic families. For example, adoption is inconsistent with the traditions of African American families (Burnette, 1997). Adopting one's own grandchildren changes the family structure and also denies the biological parent a role within the family. The termination of parental rights also ends the opportunity for the caregiver to become a grandparent to the child again. All of these assumptions can create problematic situations for grandparents, and can compromise functioning and relationships within the family system.

CONCLUSION

Examining custodial grandparents using a diversity perspective provides an understanding of ways that the profession of social work can be more responsive to the experiences of these caregivers. From a practice perspective, support groups have been a primary method of providing information and social support. However, the diversity within the population needs to be a part of assessing the structure and composition of the group. An assessment of the age, gender, and community type (e.g., rural, urban) will provide the facilitators with a beginning point to understand some of the issues that grandparents face.

In addition, a better theoretical understanding of grandparents is needed to guide practice. Information about transitions and risk junctures that might have particular meaning for diverse families is needed to understand the dynamic quality of life (Kropf & Wilks, 2003). For example, the current cohort of African American grandparents may have experienced segregated classrooms when they were enrolled as students. Their experience with educational institutions may impact their current understanding and participation with their grandchildren's school. Teachers, school social workers, and other educational personnel need to be sensitive to these issues when working with grandparents. Other junctures or risk situations may include late childhood/adolescence, where experimentation with drugs or sexual behaviors may begin. Work with families at this critical phase may help families from averting crises in functioning.

The diversity of grandparents who provide care also impacts policy-related issues of kinship care. Due to the various connotations of "family," grandparents who are raising grandchildren may or may not be interested in formalizing their caregiving relationship. While various forms of formalized care exist, grandparents may find themselves in the position of pursuing actions that are antithetical to their beliefs about family systems. Adoption is a prime example where formal ties between biological parent and child are severed. For families of color, especially African American families that have an historic experience with separation of family members, this option may be culturally dystonic. Policies that diminish families' sense of their loyalties and bonds need to be reexamined in light of a more multicultural framework.

Finally, implications for social work education are also apparent. Content on grandparent-headed families can be infused in several places of the curriculum (Kropf & Burnette, 2003; Kropf & Wilks, 2003). Teaching strategies that provide students with an opportunity to learn about diversity within this population include the use of case studies that compare the experience between families from diverse racial backgrounds, specifically addressing the strengths and resilience that are evident. Other instructional strategies include service learning which is a type of community service that promotes both student develpment and community goals (Gray, Ondaatje, & Zakaras, 1999). Examples of service learning projects could be a "grandparents day" in a school setting or a community-based aging service, or a resource directory for grandparents who are raising grandchildren. These instructional methods provide students with a way of broadening their conceptualization of "family," and sensitize them to the diversity within this population of grandparents who are raising their grandchildren.

REFERENCES

Albert, R. (2000). Legal issues for custodial grandparents. In B. Hayslip & R. Goldberg -Glen (Eds.). *Grandparents rasing grandchildren: Theoretical, empirical, and clinical perspectives* (pp. 327-340). New York, NY: Springer.

Anderson, G. R. (1990). Children and aids: Crisis for caregivers. In G. R. Anderson (Ed.). *Courage to care: Responding to the crisis of children with AIDS* (pp. 1-16). Washington, DC: Child Welfare League of America.

Baird, A., John, R., & Hayslip, B. (2000). Custodial grandparents among African Americans: A focus group perspective. In B. Hayslip, Jr. & R. Goldberg-Glen (Eds.). *Grandparents raising grandchildren: Theoretical, empirical, and clinical perspectives* (pp. 125-144). New York, NY: Springer.

Baydar, N., & Brooks-Gunn, J. (1998). Profiles of grandmothers who help care for their grandchildren in the United States. *Family Relations, 47,* 385-393.

Bowers, B. F., & Myers, B. J. (1999). Grandmothers providing care for grandchildren: Consequences of various levels of caregiving. *Family Relations, 48,* 303-311.

Brown, D. R., & Boyce-Mathis, A. (2000). Surrogate parenting across generations: African American women caring for a child with special needs. *Journal of Mental Health and Aging, 6,* 339-351.

Burnette, D. (1999). Social relationships of Latino grandparent caregivers: A role theory perspective. *The Gerontologist, 39,* 49-58.

Burnette, D. (1998). Grandparents rearing grandchildren: A school-based small group intervention. *Research on Social Work Practice, 8,* 10-27.

Burnette, D. (1997). Grandparents raising grandchildren in the inner city. *Families In Society, 78,* 489-501.

Burton, L. M. (1992). Black grandparents rearing children of drug-addicted parents: Stressors, outcomes, and social service needs. *The Gerontologist, 32,* 744-751.

Burton, L. M. (1996). Age norms, the timing of family role transitions, and intergenerational caregiving among aging African American women. *The Gerontologist, 36,* 199-208.

Burton, L. M., & Dilworth-Anderson, P. (1991). The intergenerational family roles of aged Black Americans. *Marriage and Family Review, 16,* 311-330.

Caliandro, G., & Hughes, C. (1998). The experience of being a grandmother who is the primary caregiver for her HIV positive grandchild. *Nursing Research, 47,* 107-113.

Caputo, R. K. (1999). Grandmothers and coresident grandchildren. *Families in Society, 80,* 120-126.

Chalfie, D. (1994). *Going it alone: A closer look at grandparents parenting grandchildren.* Washington DC: American Association of Retired Persons.

Chenoweth, L. (2000). Grandparent education. In B. Hayslip & R. Goldberg-Glen (Eds.). *Grandparents raising grandchildren: Theoretical, empirical, and clinical perspectives* (pp. 307-326). New York, NY: Springer.

Cox, C. (2002). Empowering African American custodial grandparents. *Social Work, 47,* 45-54.

Cox, C., Brooks, L., & Valcarcel, C. (2000). Culture and caregiving: A study of Latino grandparents. In C. Cox (Ed.). *To grandmother's house we go and stay: Perspectives on custodial grandparents* (pp. 218-232). New York, NY: Springer.

Crumbley J., & Little, R. (Eds.) (1997). *Relatives raising children: An overview of kinship care.* Washington, DC: Child Welfare League of America.

Dressel, P. L., & Barnhill, S. K. (1994). Reframing gerontological thought and practice: The case of grandmothers with daughters in prison. *The Gerontologist, 34,* 685-691.

Dubowitz, H., Feigelman, S., Harrington, D., Starr, R., Jr., & Zuravin, S. (1994). Children in kinship care: How do they fare. *Children and Youth Services Review, 16,* 85-106.

Emick, M. A., & Hayslip, B., Jr. (1999). Custodial grandparenting: Stresses, coping skills, and relationships with grandchildren. *International Journal of Human Development, 48*(1), 35-61.

Flint, M., & Perez-Porter, M. (1997). Grandparent caregivers: Legal and economic issues. *Journal of Gerontological Social Work, 28* (1/2), 63-76.

Force, L. T., Botsford, A., Pisano, P. A., & Holbert, A. (2000). Grandparents raising children with and without a developmental disability: Preliminary comparisons. *Journal of Gerontological Social Work, 33,* 5-21.

Fuller-Thomson, E., & Minkler, M. (2000). Mental and physical health of grandparents raising their grandchildren. *Journal of Mental Health and Aging, 6,* 311-323.

Fuller-Thomson, E., Minkler, M., & Driver, D. (1997). A profile of grandparents raising grandchildren in the United States. *The Gerontologist, 37,* 406-411.

Generations United (1999). *Fact sheet: Grandparents and other relatives raising children: Challenges of caring for the second family.*

Goodman, C., & Silverstein, M. (2002). Grandmothers raising grandchildren: Family structure and well-being in culturally diverse families. *The Gerontologist, 42,* 676-689.

Gray, M. J., Ondaatje, E. H., & Zakaras, L. (1999). *Combining service and learning in higher education.* Santa Monica, CA: RAND Corp.

Hayslip, B., Shore, J., & Henderson, C. E. (2000). Perceptions of grandparents' influence in the lives of their grandchildren. In B. Hayslip & R. Goldberg-Glen (Eds.). *Grandparents raising grandchildren: Theoretical, empirical, and clinical perspectives* (pp. 35-46). New York, NY: Springer.

Hayslip, B., Shore, J., Henderson, C. E., & Lambert, P. R. (1998). Custodial grandparenting and the impact of grandchildren with problems on role satisfaction and role meaning. *Journals of Gerontology Series B: Psychological Sciences and Social Sciences, 53*B(3), s164-s173.

Hunter, A. G., & Taylor, R. J. (1998). Grandparenthood in African American families. In M. E. Szinovacz (Ed.), *Handbook on grandparenthood* (pp. 70-86). Westport, CT: Greenwood.

Ingram, C. (1996). Kinship care as a child welfare service. In R. L. Hegar & M. Scannapieco (Eds.). *Kinship foster care: Policy, practice, and research.* (pp. 28-53). New York: Oxford University Press.

Janicki, M. P., McCallion, P., Grant-Griffin, L., & Kolomer, S. R. (2000). Grandparent Caregivers I: Characteristics of the grandparents and the children with disabilities they care for. *Journal of Gerontological Social Work, 33*(3), 35-56.

Jendrek, M. P. (1994). Grandparents who parent their grandchildren: Circumstances and decisions. *The Gerontologist, 34,* 206-216.

Kelley, S. J., Yorker, B. C., & Whitley, D. (1997). To grandmother's house we go . . . and stay: Children raised in intergenerational families. *Journal of Gerontological Nursing, 23*(9), 12-20.

Kelly, T. B., & Kropf, N. P. (1995). Stigmatized and perpetual parents: Older parents caring for adult children with life-long disabilities. *Journal of Gerontological Social Work, 24*(1/2), 3-16.

Kolomer, S. R. (2000). Kinship foster care and its impact on grandmother caregivers. *Journal of Gerontological Social Work, 33*(3), 85-10.

Kolomer, S. R., & McCallion, P. (Under Review). The presence of depression in grandfathers caring for their grandchildren. *International Journal of Aging and Human Development.*

Kolomer, S., McCallion, P., & Overendyer, J. (2003). Why support groups help: Successful interventions for grandparent caregivers. In B. Hayslip, & J. H. Patrick (Eds.). *Working with custodial grandparents* (pp. 111-126). New York: Springer.

Kolomer, S., McCallion, P., & Janicki, M. (2002). African-American grandmother carers of children with disabilities: Predictors of depressive symptoms. *Journal of Gerontological Social Work, 37* (3/4), 45-64.

Kropf, N. P. (1997). Older parents of adults with developmental disabilities: Practice issues and service needs. *Journal of Family Psychotherapy, 8*(2), 35-52.

Kropf, N. P., & Burnette, D. (2003). Grandparents as family caregivers: Lessons for intergenerational education. *Educational Gerontology, 29*, 361-372.

Kropf, N. P., & Wilks, S. (2003). Grandparents raising grandchildren. In B. Berkman & L. Harootyan (Eds.). *Social work and health care in an aging world* (pp. 177-200). New York, NY: Springer.

Maluccio, A. N., Fein, E., & Olmstead, K. A. (1986). *Permanency planning for children: Concepts and methods.* New York: Tavistock.

McCallion, P., Janicki, M. P., & Grant-Griffin, L. (1997). Exploring the impact of culture and acculturation on older families caregiving for persons with developmental disabilities. *Family Relations, 46*, 347-357.

McCallion, P., Janicki, M. P., Grant-Griffin, L., & Kolomer, S. (2000). Grandparent caregivers II: Service needs and service provision issues. *Journal of Gerontological Social Work, 33*(3), 57-84.

McGowen, B. G., & Studt, E. (1991). Children in social work. In A. Gitterman (Ed.), *Handbook of social work practice with vulnerable populations.* (pp. 382-415). New York: Columbia University Press.

Michaels, D., & Levine, C. (1993). Estimates of the number of motherless youth orphaned by AIDS in the United States. *Journal of the American Medical Association, 268*, 3456-3461.

Minkler, M., & Roe, K. M. (1993). *Grandmothers as caregivers: Raising children of the crack cocaine epidemic,* Newbury Park: Sage Publications.

Minkler, M., Roe, K. M., & Price, M. (1992). The physical and emotional health of grandmothers raising grandchildren in the crack cocaine epidemic. *The Gerontologist, 32*, 752-761.

Minkler, M., Roe, K. M., & Robertson-Beckley, R. J. (1994). Raising grandchildren from crack cocaine households: Effects on family and friendship ties of African-American women. *American Journal of Orthopsychiatry, 64*, 20-29.

Musil, C. M. (1998). Health, stress, coping, and social support in grandmother caregivers. *Health Care for Women International, 19*, 441-455.

Myers, L., Kropf, N. P., & Robinson, M. M. (2002). Grandparents raising grandchildren: Case management in a rural setting. *Journal of Human Behavior in the Social Environment, 5*(1), 53-71.

Pebley, A. R., & Rudkin, L. L. (1999). Grandparents caring for grandchildren: What do we know? *Journal of Family Issues, 20*, 218-242.

Phillips, S., & Bloom, B. (1998). In whose best interest? The impact of changing public policy on relatives caring for children with incarcerated parents. *Child Welfare, 77*(5), 531-541.

Pinson-Milburn, N. M., Fabian, E. S., Schlossberg, N. K., & Pyle, M. (1996). Grandparents raising grandchildren. *Journal of Counseling and Development, 74*, 548-554.

Poindexter, C. P., & Linsk, N. L. (1999). "I'm just glad that I'm here": Stories of seven African American HIV-affected grandmothers. *Journal of Gerontological Social Work, 32*, 63-81.

Pruchno, R. (1999). Raising grandchildren: The experience of Black and White grandmothers. *The Gerontologist, 39*, 209-221.

Pruchno, R., & McKenney, D. (2000). The effects of custodial and co-resident households on the mental health of grandmothers. *Journal of Mental Health and Aging, 6*, 291-310.

Robinson, M. M., & Kropf, N. P. (2001). Pathways into care for rural custodial grandparents. Paper presented at the Annual Program Meeting of the Council on Social Work Education. Nashville, TN.

Robinson, M. M., Kropf, N. P., & Myers, L. (2000). Grandparents raising grandchildren in rural communities. *Journal of Aging and Mental Health, 6*, 353-365.

Roe, K. M., Minkler, M., Saunders, F., & Thomson, G. E. (1996). Health of grandmothers raising children of the crack cocaine epidemic. *Med Care, 34*(11), 1072-1084.

Silverstein, N. M., & Vehvilainen, L. (1998). *Raising awareness about grandparents raising grandchildren in Massachusetts.* University of Massachusetts, Boston MA: Gerontology Institute.

Strawbridge, W. M., Wallhagen, J. I., Shema, S. J., & Kaplan, G. A. (1997). New burdens or more of the same? Comparing grandparent, spouse, and adult-child caregivers. *The Gerontologist, 37*(4), 505-510.

Strom, R. D., & Strom, S. K. (1993). Grandparents raising grandchildren: Goals and support groups. *Educational Gerontology, 19*, 705-715.

Szinovacz, M. E., DeViney. S., & Atkinson, M. P. (1999). Effects of surrogate parenting on grandparents' well-being. *Journal of Gerontology: Social Sciences, 54B*(6), S376-388.

Wabanki Legal News (2002). *www.ptla.org/wabanaki/icwa.htm.* Indian Child Welfare Act Update.

Racial and Ethnic Differences in Family Caregiving in California

Nancy Giunta
Julian Chow
Andrew E. Scharlach
Teresa S. Dal Santo

SUMMARY. Family caregivers are the main source of long-term care for older persons in the United States. At the same time, cultural values and beliefs shape decisions surrounding who provides care and whether families use formal support interventions to assist the caregiver. The

---

Nancy Giunta, MSW, MA, is a doctoral student, University of California at Berkeley, School of Social Welfare and Graduate Research Associate at the Center for the Advanced Study of Aging Services. Julian Chow, PhD, is Associate Professor of Social Welfare at the University of California at Berkeley. Andrew E. Scharlach, PhD, is Director, Center for the Advanced Study of Aging Services and Professor of Social Welfare, University of California at Berkeley, where he holds the Eugene and Rose Kleiner Chair in Aging. Teresa S. Dal Santo, PhD, Senior Research Associate, serves as Project Director for the current study, conducted to help implement and evaluate the National Family Caregiver Support Program in California.

Address correspondence to: Nancy Giunta, Center for the Advanced Study of Aging Services, University of California at Berkeley, 120 Haviland Hall, #7400, Berkeley, CA 94720-7400 (E-mail: n_joonta@yahoo.com).

The current study was conducted under an inter-agency agreement with the California Department of Aging. The authors thank Wei Li for his work on the statistical analysis for this paper. The authors also wish to thank the anonymous reviewers of an earlier draft, whose comments helped improve the overall clarity of this article.

[Haworth co-indexing entry note]: "Racial and Ethnic Differences in Family Caregiving in California." Giunta, Nancy et al. Co-published simultaneously in *Journal of Human Behavior in the Social Environment* (The Haworth Social Work Practice Press, an imprint of The Haworth Press, Inc.) Vol. 9, No. 4, 2004, pp. 85-109; and: *Diversity and Aging in the Social Environment* (eds: Sherry M. Cummings, and Colleen Galambos) The Haworth Social Work Practice Press, an imprint of The Haworth Press, Inc., 2004, pp. 85-109; Single or multiple copies of this article are available for a fee from The Haworth Document Delivery Service [1-800-HAWORTH, 9:00 a.m. - 5:00 p.m. (EST). E-mail address: docdelivery@haworthpress.com].

http://www.haworthpress.com/web/JHBSE
Digital Object Identifier: 10.1300/J137v09n04_05

current article examines how the family caregiving experience differs among racial and ethnic groups in terms of caregiver characteristics, service utilization, caregiver strain, and coping mechanisms. Telephone interviews were conducted in English and Spanish with a random sample of 1,643 respondents in California who provide care to someone age 50 or over. Bivariate analyses showed evidence of ethnic differences in the demographic characteristics of caregivers, intensity of care provided, caregiver health, level of financial strain, religious service attendance, formal service utilization and barriers to formal services. Odds ratios showed that White and African American caregivers were about two times as likely to use formal caregiver services as were Asian/Native Hawaiian/Pacific Islander and Latina American caregivers. Implied by these findings is the need for further understanding of caregiver service needs among diverse racial and ethnic groups. *[Article copies available for a fee from The Haworth Document Delivery Service: 1-800-HAWORTH. E-mail address: <docdelivery@haworthpress.com> Website: <http://www. HaworthPress.com> © 2004 by The Haworth Press, Inc. All rights reserved.]*

KEYWORDS. Caregiving, ethnic differences, formal service use

INTRODUCTION

While the overall population of Americans age 65 and over is projected to double by the year 2050, the percentage of racial and ethnic minority elders will increase at a much higher rate during this time (U.S. Bureau of the Census, 2000). From 2000 to 2050, projections indicate that the African American elderly population will quadruple; the Hispanic elderly population will grow to seven times its current size; the Asian/Pacific Islander elderly population will increase to 6.5 times its current size; and American Indian elderly will increase to 3.5 times their current numbers (U.S. Bureau of the Census, 2000).

Family caregivers are the main source of long-term care for older persons in this country (Liu, Manton, & Aragon, 2000). Approximately 75% of frail or disabled elderly adults are cared for at home or in the community by family members or other informal care providers (Bengtson, Rosenthal, & Burton, 1996; Liu & Manton, 1994; Mui, Choi, & Monk, 1998). Research to date has captured many aspects of family caregiving and has demonstrated that the availability of family members to provide care tends to be a major factor predicting whether or not a disabled elderly person will remain at home or be institutionalized (Scharlach & Greenlee, 2001). In order to help support family caregivers in their role, it is important to understand caregivers demand for formal and informal support and caregivers experiences in trying to meet this demand. This increased understanding of caregiver needs and demand across an increasingly racially and ethnically diverse population will serve to clarify and enrich the picture for policy development and program implementation.

The current article examines how the family caregiving experience, including formal service use, differs among racial and ethnic groups. Family caregiving is provided in a context in which cultural values and beliefs shape decisions around who gives care and who uses formal support interventions. For service providers, the ability to provide relevant and meaningful interventions that address the diverse needs of caregivers requires an understanding of this cultural context, including social class, religious beliefs and practices, as well as views of the aging process, wellness, and disease. In developing interventions for ethnic minority elders with dementia and their caregivers, Gallagher-Thompson et al. (2003) point out that it is necessary to implement culturally sensitive interventions that incorporate caregivers' values and beliefs.

One can conceptualize the influence of race and ethnicity on the family caregiving experience through a framework such as Andersen and Newman's model of health behavior and service utilization (Andersen & Newman, 1973; Andersen, 1995). This model, used extensively in the health and social service literature, has been shown to predict formal service utilization. The behavioral model consists of predisposing, enabling, and need variables that together explain and predict service use. Predisposing variables include demographic characteristics and health beliefs people have that might influence a perceived need for health services (Andersen, 1995). Enabling variables consist of personal and community resources available to an individual that either facilitate service accessibility or create barriers to services. Such enabling variables include the level of strain experienced in the caregiving role, the knowledge of available services, or the existence of barriers to services. Finally, the need factor, perhaps the strongest predictor of service use in the model, consists of an individual's perceived need for service (Calsyn & Winter, 2000; Yeatts, Crow, & Folts, 1992).

Using the behavioral model of health services as a conceptual framework, we view a caregiver's race and ethnicity as a predisposing factor, which may influence other predisposing or enabling factors that impact a caregiver's perceived need for, and therefore, utilization of services.

Enabling factors that may be influenced by race and ethnicity include the availability of culturally appropriate and affordable services, the use of family or other informal networks to assist the caregiver, the caregiver's perception of his or her role, and the level of strain or burden experienced through this role. There is mixed evidence that race and ethnicity play a significant role in the family caregiving experience in terms of caregiver characteristics, the perception of strain and coping within the caregiver role, and formal service utilization (Dilworth-Anderson, Williams, & Gibson, 2002; Connell & Gibson, 1997; Janevic & Connell, 2001).

Caregiver Characteristics

Much of the research on ethnic differences among caregiver support systems has focused on comparing Whites with one ethnic group, most often African Americans (Ajrouch, Antonucci, & Janevic, 2001; Connell & Gibson, 1997; Dilworth-Anderson et al., 2002). Connell and Gibson reviewed 12 studies for the purpose of exploring the effects of race, culture and ethnicity on caregiving. Most studies in their review compared White and African American caregivers (10 of 12), while one study compared White and Hispanic caregivers and one study compared Hispanic and African American caregivers. Overall, they found that non-White caregivers: (1) were less likely to be a spouse and more likely to be an adult child, friend, or other family member, (2) expressed stronger beliefs of filial support, (3) reported lower levels of caregiver stress, and (4) were more likely to use religion, prayer, or faith as a coping strategy (Connell & Gibson, 1997). In addition, African American caregivers have been found to perform more intensive caregiving activities and care for persons with greater functional impairment than White caregivers (Navaie-Waliser et al., 2001).

Strain and Coping

Caregiver burden and other measures of strain, including depression, tend to be higher among White and Hispanic caregivers than among African American caregivers (Connell & Gibson, 1997; Dilworth-Anderson et al., 2002; Mui, Choi, & Monk, 1998). These differences have been attributed to a more positive perception of the caregiving role among African Americans (Janevic & Connell, 2001), and the higher likelihood of using religious activities as a means of coping (Navaie-Waliser et al., 2001). In order to understand the current state of research on caregiving among diverse groups, Dilworth-Anderson, Williams, & Brent (2002) conducted an extensive review and synthesis of the literature. In regards to coping, they linked higher levels of spirituality and religiosity with lower measures of depression and burden. Further, the use of different coping strategies such as appraisal of the situation by African American caregivers led to different levels of depression and burden when compared with White caregivers. The role of culture can be linked to methods of coping and appraisal of the caregiver situation, while findings on cultural values, norms, expectations, and feelings of obligation and reciprocity have shown that these factors may encourage a positive self-appraisal of the ethnic minority caregiver in his or her role of providing care for an elder.

Service Utilization

The majority of existing evidence suggests that ethnic minority caregivers use more informal than formal support, with informal support being provided by close as well as distant family members (Aranda & Knight, 1997; Connell & Gibson, 1997; Dilworth-Anderson et al., 2002; Mui, Choi, & Monk, 1998). Upon examining both formal and informal support, Dilworth-Anderson and colleagues found that informal support among White caregivers is more likely to consist only of immediate family when compared with minority caregivers, who tend to have more diverse informal networks.

Minority caregivers express a greater need for formal support services than do White caregivers, and have been shown to benefit from those services; however, most research has found that minority caregivers tend to use formal support services utilization, found that White elders (both caregivers and substantially less than their White counterparts (Dilworth-Anderson et al., 2002; Dunlop, Manheim, Song, & Chang, 2002; Tennstedt & Chang, 1998; White-Means & Thornton, 1996). Mui and her colleagues (1998), for example, using the Andersen model of health service care recipients) were significantly more likely to use formal services than both Hispanic and African American elders. One exception is a recent study by Toseland, McCallion, Gerber, & Banks (2002), which found that being non-White was associated with increased human service use among caregivers of persons with dementia. These mixed findings clearly indicate there is a need to further explore service use among ethnically diverse caregivers.

Barriers to Service

Empirical work examining formal service use by minority elders is growing, but as Mui et al. (1998) observe, "reasons for their persistent underutilization are not well-known or understood" (p. 104). Dilworth-Anderson et al. (2002) found that caregivers of older ethnic minorities rarely used formal services and hypothesized that this non-service use may be due to: (a) shame, (b) feelings of obligation, or (c) lack of culturally sensitive formal services. Other barriers to service utilization among ethnic and racial minorities may include lack of transportation, lack of knowledge about services, cost of services, language barriers, negative perception of services, or negative prior experience with services due to cultural insensitivity (Damskey, 2000; Mui, Choi, & Monk, 1998).

The Present Study

The present study examines racial and ethnic variations among family caregivers in California. California provides a particularly interesting and useful environment in which to examine ethnic differences in the caregiving role. First, California has the largest and most diverse older adult population of any state within the U.S. According to 2000 census data, close to 3.6 million Californians were 65 years of age and older, of whom approximately 70% were White, 13% were Hispanic or Latina, 10% were Asian, 5% were Black, and 2% were of another or multiracial identity (U.S. Census Bureau, 2000). Moreover, more than 1.5 million adults in California have physical or mental disabilities necessitating ongoing assistance with day-to-day activities (GAO, 1995). Second, it is estimated that close to 16% of households in California are involved in providing care to someone age 50 or older (Scharlach, Sirotnik et al., 2003), which is comparable to a 1997 national study indicating that approximately 17% of all U.S. households with a telephone contain at least one caregiver (National Alliance for Caregiving and the American Association of Retired Persons, 1997). Third, California has a well-established array of potential resources for caregivers, offered through a broad range of public and private service providers, including religious, social, and health care organizations. Of particular note are California's Caregiver Resource Centers (CRCs), a statewide network of 11 regional centers assisting caregivers. Finally, California's aging network as a whole is well-developed, including 33 AAAs (15 of which are co-located with county governments), multiple chapters of the Alzheimer's Association, Alzheimer's Day Care Resource Centers, pub-licly-funded case management programs, and community-based pro-grams provided by non-governmental organizations. The existence of a broad service network allows us to give particular attention to service use and needs among caregivers: who uses and does not use services; what barriers exist that prevent service access; and, in addition to exist-ing services, what could be offered to assist family caregivers in a more culturally sensitive and equitable manner.

This exploratory study examines racial and ethnic variations among caregivers with regard to: caregiver characteristics, caregiver strain and coping activities, service utilization patterns, and potential barriers to service. Using a sampling method more rigorous than previous studies, the probability sample used in this study is highly representative of caregiving households in California and includes several racial/ethnic categories often neglected in prior studies. While the current study does not specifically measure cultural values, it provides a descriptive analy-sis using a highly representative sample from which patterns of service use and non-use may be identified, that will add substantially to knowl-edge regarding the family caregiving experience across cultures. Fur-thermore, this study can be used to assist policymakers and practitioners to design new programs that are more inclusive, culturally sensitive, and appropriate in meeting a wide variety of informal as well as formal caregiver needs.

METHODOLOGY

Design

Data for this study were gathered through a household survey of Cali-fornia caregivers conducted as part of an interagency agreement be-tween the California Department of Aging and the Center for the Advanced Study of Aging Services at the University of California, Berkeley. The initial statewide sampling frame consisted of telephone numbers reflective of households with phones throughout California, which were sorted into working blocks of 100 contiguous numbers, then randomly sampled within working blocks. To ensure that some un-listed phone numbers were included in the sample, the original list was supplemented by using a working number as a seed number from which one other number was generated by adding a constant. Telephone inter-views were conducted between March 28 and August 22, 2002 from the facilities of California State University, San Bernardino's Institute of Applied Research and Policy Analysis using computer-assisted telephone interviewing (CATI) equipment and software. Caregiver screening questions and interviews were conducted in English and Spanish.

Two screening questions, asked in either English or Spanish, were used to identify a caregiver of an adult age 50 or over. The first question read: "Do you or does anyone in your household currently provide assistance or support to an adult relative or friend who is ill, disabled, or elderly?" "Assistance or support" was defined within the introduction as providing assistance for at least a couple of hours a month with personal needs, household chores, taking care of finances, or arranging for outside services. The second screening question asked the ages (and relationships) of the people for whom the respondent provides care, thus enabling the interviewer to identify the target population: caregivers of adults age 50 or over.

Questionnaire construction. The questionnaire was constructed to elicit information in six areas: the demographic characteristics of caregivers and care recipients; care recipient health and functioning; level of care provided by the caregiver; assistance required by the care recipient; services provided to caregiver, and unmet needs of the caregiver; and impact of caregiving on work, emotional health, and physical health.

Demographic characteristics included age, gender, race/ethnicity (using U.S. Census 2000 categories), educational attainment, type of relationship, country of origin, living arrangement, and distance between caregiver and care recipient, reported by the caregiver as the time it takes to travel between caregiver and care recipient residences. A measure of care recipient health and functioning consisted of a checklist of physical and mental illnesses presented to the caregiver to report whether or not the care recipient had any of the conditions. The level of care provided by the caregiver and assistance required by the care recipient were determined by asking the respondent whether the care recipient needed assistance with any of six ADL and IADL activities, and whether the assistance was provided by the caregiver, family or friends, or paid service providers.

To determine formal and informal support utilized by the caregiver as well as unmet needs of the caregiver, the respondent was asked if he or she used a list of common caregiver services. If the caregiver indicated that a service was used, he or she was asked whether the service was provided by formal (community agency) or informal (family or friends) sources. To measure barriers to service use, the respondent was presented with a list of possible reasons he or she had not received "more outside help" caring for the care recipient and was asked whether or not each reason applied to his or her situation. Three separate single-item Likert scales were used to determine emotional, physical, and financial strain experienced by caregivers. Caregiver health was measured with a self-reported health question in addition to a question asking caregivers whether they experienced any physical or mental health conditions which made it difficult to provide assistance or support to the care recipients. Five questions adapted from the Cultural Justifications Caregiving Scale (Dilworth-Anderson, 1995) were used to explore the appraisal of the caregiving experience and the effects of the caregiving situation on the family. See the Appendix for selected examples of survey questions.

Sample

The final sample consisted of 1,643 individuals who were providing care to someone age 50 or over. This sample size yielded an accuracy rate of plus/minus approximately 2.4% at a 95% level of confidence. One in six households was found to contain at least one caregiver, comparable to national estimates that approximately 17% of all U.S. households with a telephone contain at least one caregiver (National Alliance for Caregiving and the American Association of Retired Persons, 1997). Ninety-eight interviews were conducted in Spanish and the remaining 1,545 were conducted in English.

The survey was completed by 19% of identified caregivers. Although a 19% response rate appears low, it is consistent with the response rates of a similar study (National Alliance for Caregiving and American Association of Retired Persons, 1997). The response rate reflects the calculated tradeoff between response rate, richness of data, and length and complexity of the questionnaire (mean length = 25.4 minutes).

To help determine whether the sampling reflected systematic bias, two analyses were conducted. First, the ethnicity of all households contacted was compared with general California figures for individuals and households. Second, we compared the ethnicity of our sample with projections of the ethnicity of California caregivers based on a national study (National Alliance for Caregiving and the American Association of Retired Persons, 1997). The results of these analyses provide supporting evidence that the sample was relatively representative of the California population as a whole, individually and by household, and the population of caregivers, despite the slight over-representation of

Latino/Hispanic and under-representation of Asian/Pacific Islander caregivers, as shown in Table 1.

The racial/ethnic composition of the sample was as follows: 61% White, 25% Latino/Hispanic, 6% African American, and 5% Asian/Native Hawaiian/Pacific Islander. Overall, most of the caregivers surveyed were between 35- and 64-years-old (67%), married (60%), and did not have children under the age of 18 living at home (69%). Most caregivers were born in the United States (86%), but a notable number (6%) reported Mexico as their country of origin.

An overwhelming majority of the sample was female (75%). Most caregivers reported having graduated from high school (69%), with 35% reporting either a college degree or post-graduate education. Most caregivers had annual incomes over $30,000 (60% of those willing to reveal their income), with a significant number (36% of those willing to reveal their income) reporting incomes over $50,000. Income varied considerably by race and ethnicity, which will be discussed in subsequent sections of this article. The demographic profile of caregivers in this sample is consistent with findings from national studies (National Alliance for Caregiving and American Association of Retired Persons, 1997), taking into consideration differences that occur when comparing the more diverse California population to residents in the rest of the nation.

TABLE 1. Ethnic Distribution of California Population vs. the California Caregiver Study Sample

	General Population Over 18 (California Households)	Caregivers Caring for Person Over Age of 50 (Completed Survey)
Ethnicity		
White/ Caucasian	58%	61%
African American	7%	6%
Asian	10%	5%
American Indian/Alaska Native	0.6%	1%
Native Hawaiian/Pacific Islander	0.2%	0.2%
Latino/Hispanic	22%	25%
Other	2%	2%
Total	100%	100%

Analysis

The independent variable, caregiver race and ethnicity, was collapsed into five categories: Asian/Native Hawaiian/Pacific Islander (ANHPI), Latino/Hispanic (LAT), African American/non-Hispanic Black (AA), Caucasian/non-Hispanic White (WH), and other (OTH), consisting of American Indian/Alaska Native and those who reported their race as "mixed." Caregiver formal service utilization (CGFSU) was a composite score constructed by totaling the number of services, out of 12 possible types of service (e.g., "Have you received education or training on how to assist your [relationship]?" or "Have you received advice or counseling from a clergy person?") received within the last year from sources other than family members or friends (see Appendix for more extensive list of sample survey questions). Because the distribution of this variable was highly skewed, the variable was transformed into an ordinal variable consisting of three categories describing different levels of CGFSU: low, medium, and high. Low CGFSU consisted of no formal services used within the last year, medium CGFSU consisted of one or two formal services in the last year, and high CGFSU consisted of three or more formal services used within the last year. Once transformed into the three ordered categories, the distribution of CGFSU was more symmetrical, thus making the variable more appropriate for analysis.

Odds ratios were used to predict differences in CGFSU and differences in physical, emotional, and financial strain among the five ethnic groups. Chi-square and ANOVA tests were conducted to explore, at the bivariate level, ethnic differences among all other variables.

RESULTS

Racial/ethnic groups were compared with regard to several factors. Using the behavioral model of health service use as a framework, the factors included: predisposing variables (caregiver demographic and other characteristics such as the type of relationship between care recipient and caregiver, caregiver health and well-being), enabling variables (appraisal of the caregiving situation, including level of family conflict, positive aspects of the caregiving situation, and coping mechanisms), caregiver formal service utilization, and perceived barriers to services. Differences in self-reported health status, financial strain, perceived emotional support, religious service attendance/religiosity, formal service use, and barriers to formal services emerged across different ethnic groups.

Caregiver Characteristics

As shown in Table 2, demographic differences among caregivers by race and ethnicity included age, education level, and household income. White caregivers, with a mean age of 54 were significantly older than non-White and Hispanic caregivers, whose mean ages ranged from 44 to 49 (F = 42.9, p < .001). Asian/Native Hawaiian/Pacific Islander caregivers had the highest proportion of caregivers with any post-secondary education (81%) while Latina caregivers were least likely (25%) to have graduated from high school (X^2 = 194.4, p < .001). Latina and African American caregivers were significantly more likely to have had (53% for both groups) annual household incomes of less than $30,000 ($X^2$ = 49.1, p < .001) compared to Asian/Native Hawaiian/Pacific Islander (34%) and White caregivers (35%).

Latina and African American caregivers were significantly more likely to be caring for non-spouses such as parents or grandparents (X^2 = 50.33, p < .001) compared with other caregivers. Care recipient living arrangements also differed significantly by ethnicity. Asian/Native Hawaiian/Pacific Islander care recipients were most likely to be living with their caregivers (X^2 = 20.7, p < .001). White caregivers were least likely to have primary responsibility for children under age 18 living in the home (24%) while Latina caregivers were most likely to be responsible (47%) for children in the home (X^2 = 75.68, p < .001). Across ethnicities, caregivers were spending on average 42 hours per week (S.E. 1.64) providing assistance to their care recipients (Table 3). African American caregivers, who spent an average of 56 hours per week, and Latina caregivers, who spent 49 hours per week, were spending significantly more time each week providing assistance than White caregivers, who were providing a weekly average of 37 hours (F = 3.622, p < .01). As shown in Table 3, standard deviations for these distributions were high, which was the result of the bimodal nature of this distribution. Most caregivers (75%) were providing assistance either up to 35 hours or they were providing constant, 24-hour care (16%), with few caregivers falling between these two categories. Non-White caregivers were significantly more likely to report that they provided constant, 24-hour care compared with White caregivers (20% vs. 14%, respectively; X^2 = 10.33, p < .05).

African American caregivers (39%) were most likely to report their health as "poor" or "fair" compared with 25% of caregivers from other

TABLE 2. Caregiver Social and Demographic Characteristics, by Race and Ethnicity

	WH	LAT	ANHPI	AA	OTH
Age* (n = 1,597)	M = 54.36	M = 43.7	M = 45.2	M = 49.3	M = 49.2
	%	%	%	%	%
Under 35	20.7	34.5	26.7	28.7	32.1
35-49	24.5	26.3	28.0	27.7	22.6
50-64	26.9	23.3	33.3	24.5	20.8
65 and older	27.9	15.9	12.0	19.1	22.5
Gender (n = 1,635)					
Female	74.1	75.7	73.3	80.2	79.6
Male	25.9	24.3	26.7	19.8	20.4
Highest level of schooling* (n = 1,625)					
<HS grad	5.9	24.9	2.7	10.4	3.7
HS grad	20.0	22.9	16.2	22.9	20.4
Post HS ed. or training	35.5	28.7	18.9	39.6	42.6
College graduate	24.5	18.1	43.2	20.8	22.2
Post-grad degree	14.1	5.3	18.9	6.3	11.1
2001 Household Income* (n = 1,643)					
Under $30,000	34.8	52.7	33.9	53.2	23.9
$30,000 or more	65.3	47.3	66.1	46.8	76.1
Current marital status (n = 1,499)					
Married/partner	65.6	61.2	64.8	34.9	58.4
Separated	1.5	2.7	0	7.0	4.2
Divorced	12.1	11.7	5.6	22.1	10.4
Widowed	8.8	2.7	1.4	8.1	6.3
Never Married	11.9	21.7	28.2	27.9	20.8
Children < 18 living in household* (n = 1,630)					
Yes	23.8	47.0	41.3	35.8	33.3
No	76.2	53.0	58.7	64.2	66.7
Country of origin (n = 1,380)					
United States	96.1	67.1	33.8	96.3	88.9
Mexico	-	25.1	-	-	-
Asian/Pacific Island	-	0.3	49.2	-	-
Central America	0.2	5.5	-	2.4	-
Europe	2.4	-	-	-	2.2
Canada	0.8	-	-	-	-
Other	0.4	2.0	16.9	1.2	8.9
Relationship Type: Who is CG assisting?* (n = 1635)					
Parent	45.8	56.8	64.0	38.1	44.4
Spouse/Partner	15.1	8.1	8.0	9.3	5.6
Friend	12.6	9.8	4.0	12.4	11.1
Parent-in-law	8.5	7.0	14.7	8.2	7.4
Grandparent	6.0	10.3	4.0	13.4	9.3
Other Extended Family	4.9	4.5	2.6	10.3	7.5
Sibling	3.3	2.5	2.7	6.2	3.7
Neighbor	3.8	1.0	0	2.1	11.1

*Chi-square analyses: significant differences among ethnicities (p < .01)

TABLE 3. Amount of Time Spent Each Week Providing Assistance, by Race and Ethnicity

Caregiver Ethnicity	Mean Hours/Week	Standard Deviation	% Reporting Constant Care**
White (baseline)	37.3	56.2	13.7
African American	55.9*	63.8	22.8
Latina	48.5*	62.6	20.0
Asian/ Native Hawaiian/ Pacific Islander	46.0	63.6	18.0
Total	41.5 hours	58.8 hours	16.1 %

*p < .05 (when compared with White caregivers): ANOVA and Tukey's post-hoc.
** p < .05: Pearson Chi-square.

racial/ethnic groups (X^2 = 18.8, p < .01). The majority of all caregivers, except those in the "other" ethnic category (n = 45), reported that health conditions or emotional problems did not serve as a barrier to providing assistance. Those caregivers in the "other" ethnicity category were significantly more likely to report that illnesses, health conditions or emotional barriers made it difficult to provide assistance to their care recipients (X^2 = 17.87, p < .01).

Caregiver Strain and Coping

Among the three types of caregiver strain measured, financial strain was the only type of strain to differ by ethnicity. As Table 4 illustrates, odds ratios showed that non-White caregivers were nearly twice as likely to report financial strain as White caregivers.

Differences in coping mechanisms emerged (Table 5) by race and ethnicity. Although the majority of all caregiver groups (77.7%) reported having someone to go to for support and understanding, White caregivers were significantly more likely to report having this emotional support than non-White caregivers (81% vs. 72%, X^2 = 18.99, p < .01). Caregivers tended to report religious service attendance either "at least once a week" or "never," with African American caregivers exhibiting the highest proportion (92.6%) of those ever attending (X^2 = 56.4, p < .001), compared with the two-thirds of non-African American caregivers ever attending religious services. The majority of all caregivers reported praying or meditating everyday, but the proportion of White and Asian/Native Hawaiian/Pacific Islander caregivers praying or meditating was significantly lower (87%) than other caregiver groups, ranging from 91 to 97% (X^2 = 42.25, p < .01).

TABLE 4. Odds Ratios Predicting Strain Among Caregivers

Caregiver Ethnicity (Baseline = White)	Mean Odds Ratio	Lower -Upper Bound	P-value
Financial Strain			
African American	2.382	1.568-3.618	<.001
Asian/ Native Hawaiian/ Pacific Islander	2.312	1.446-3.691	<.001
Latina	1.775	1.397-2.259	<.001
Emotional Strain			
African American	1.278	−1.184-1.931	Ns
Asian/ Native Hawaiian/ Pacific Islander	−1.033	−1.623-1.52	Ns
Latina	1.183	−1.063-1.489	Ns
Physical Strain			
African American	1.278	−1.184-1.931	Ns
Asian/ Native Hawaiian/ Pacific Islander	1.071	−1.492-1.713	Ns
Latina	1.183	−1.063-1.489	Ns

TABLE 5. Coping Mechanisms Reported by Caregivers by Race/Ethnicity

	All CGs	WH	LAT	ANHPI	AA	OTH
				% Yes		
Emotional Support						
Has someone to go to for support and understanding**	77.7	81.3	72.3	72.7	76.5	62.2
Religious Practices						
Attend service at least once/week**	43.0	39.9	45.1	40.9	69.1	40
Never attend religious service**	28.4	32.6	22.8	25.8	7.4	37.8
Meditate or pray at least once/week**	78.9	76.5	81.0	76.9	95.0	77.8
Never meditate or pray on own**	11.2	13.0	8.7	13.8	2.5	8.9
Perception of CG Situation			% "very much" or "somewhat"			
Making a family contribution	90.4	88.9	93.5	93.7	92.3	85.4
Setting an example for children	91.0	90.5	90.8	93.1	97.3	87.2
Has brought the family close together*	63.8	60.5	68.9	74.6	63.1	73.1
CG situation has created conflicts or disagreements in family	29.8	27.6	34.9	33.3	23.1	35.7
CG situation is a hardship for family	36.2	28.0	38.8	43.8	31.3	35.7

*p < .05, **p < .01

When asked about the positive aspects of caregiving and effects of the caregiving situation on the family, caregiver responses were mostly similar across racial/ethnic groups. Overall, nine out of 10 (90.4%) careg ivers felt they were making a contribution to their families either "very much" (68.8%) or "somewhat" (21.6%) by providing care. Most caregivers (91.0%) also felt that they were setting an example for the children in their families. Asian/Native Hawaiian/Pacific Islander caregivers were significantly more likely to report that the caregiving situation had brought their families closer together either "somewhat" or "very much," compared with all other groups (74.6% vs. 63%, X^2 = 23.42, p < .05). A minority of caregivers of all ethnicities reported that the caregiving situation created conflict "somewhat" or "very much" (29.8%). There also were no significant racial or ethnic differences among caregivers (36.2%) who claimed that caregiving was a hardship on the family either "somewhat" or "very much."

Service Utilization

Formal caregiver service utilization significantly differed by ethnicity, as African American and White caregivers were significantly more likely to use formal services than Latina or Asian/Native Hawaiian/Pacific Islander counterparts. Odds ratios predicted that African American caregivers were 1.9 times more likely to use formal services than Latina caregivers and 2.6 times more likely to use formal services than caregivers of Asian/Native Hawaiian/Pacific Islander descent. Odds ratios similarly predicted that White caregivers were more likely to use formal services than both Latina and Asian/Native Hawaiian/Pacific Islander caregivers (1.5 times and 1.9 times respectively). The implications of this finding are particularly relevant for planning culturally competent services as questions around culture and country of origin begin to emerge.

Barriers to Service Utilization

The reason most often provided for not utilizing formal service was the caregiver having all the help she or he needed, which was significantly more likely the case for White (75%) and Asian/Native Hawaiian/Pacific Islander (69%) caregivers (X^2 = 24.21, p < .001) than for Latina or African American caregivers (63% each). Although most caregivers felt they were receiving all of the formal help they needed, differences in service barriers were still identified, as shown in Table 6. Overall,

Latina and African American caregivers reported a higher number of barriers than did their White and Asian/Native Hawaiian/Pacific Islander counterparts. Latina and African American caregivers were more likely than other groups to report barriers related to poor service quality (14.5% and 15.6%, respectively, $X^2 = 31.08$, p < .01), cost (19.7% and 18.3%, respectively, $X^2 = 14.98$, p < .01), services not being available at times needed (14.4% and 13.0%, respectively, $X^2 = 18.3$, p < .01), and services not being offered by "people like you" (8.9% and 11.2%, respectively, $X^2 = 10.41$, p < .05). Asian/Native Hawaiian/Pacific Islander and Latina (11.0% and 9.3%) caregivers were more likely to report language as a barrier to formal service utilization than other groups ($X^2 = 33.51$, p < .001). Caregivers did not differ by race or ethnicity with regard to other reasons for not using services: the care recipient not wanting the service, no one to stay with the care recipient while the caregiver seeks services, lack of time for the caregiver to seek services for herself, or lack of transportation.

DISCUSSION

The purpose of this study was to examine racial and ethnic differences among caregivers. In addition to differences in formal service uti-

TABLE 6. Reasons for Not Receiving Services, by Race and Ethnicity

	All CGs	WH	LAT	ANHPI	AA	OTH
Already have help**	70.7%	75.4%	63.2%	69.2%	63.0%	57.8%
Cost**	15.7	13.5	19.7	10.6	18.3	26.9
CR doesn't want it	13.2	11.9	15.4	13.7	13.8	20.8
Services not available**	11.1	8.5	16.2	8.5	12.9	20.0
Poor service quality**	9.2	6.3	14.5	5.8	15.6	18.0
Not available at times needed**	8.8	5.8	14.4	7.1	13.0	15.7
No one to stay with CR while CG gets help	8.2	7.0	10.9	5.6	8.4	14.8
CG has no time to get help for self	8.0	7.2	8.4	12.0	6.3	17.0
Transportation not available	7.4	6.5	8.8	9.7	5.2	15.1
Services not offered by "people who are like" CG*	6.9	5.4	8.9	5.6	11.2	12.0
Language**	4.8	2.6	9.3	11.0	4.3	5.9

* p < .05 ** p < .01

lization, racial and ethnic differences were found in the demographic characteristics of caregivers, intensity of care provided, level of financial strain, and barriers to formal services. Similarities within the caregiver experience that transcended race and ethnicity included feelings around family unity, family contribution, and emotional strain.

The findings presented in this study partly support previous findings that minority caregivers have more intensive caregiving responsibilities and use fewer formal services to assist them. In addition to the greater likelihood of caring for children as well as elders, Latina and African American caregivers reported spending more hours each week providing care to their family members, who were more likely to be their parents or grandparents in old age. The fact that a high proportion of African American caregivers self-reported their health as poor raises serious concern for the well-being of both the caregivers and the care recipients in situations with such demanding roles.

The significantly lower levels of formal service use among Asian/ Native Hawaiian/Pacific Islander and Latina caregivers support previous evidence in the literature that minority caregivers tend to use fewer formal services, but raises two questions. First, considering the higher intensity of caregiving provided by these caregivers, why do they report such low levels of service use? Second, why are African American caregivers excluded from this group of low service users, considering their caregiving responsibilities are as intense as other minority groups? The common characteristics of Asian/Native Hawaiian/Pacific Islander and Latina caregivers include their greater likelihood of experiencing language as a barrier to service use compared with African American and White caregivers. This suggests that the key barrier to service use among minority caregivers may be the lack of culturally appropriate services, including services that are language specific. Considering previous evidence that minority caregivers benefit from formal service use once it is received, we must identify and eliminate the service barriers that face minority caregivers.

Although African American caregivers were more likely than other ethnic minority groups to use formal services, they also tended to report barriers to services such as poor quality of the services they received and services not being available at times they needed them. In addition, financial strain appeared to be a key factor commonly experienced by most African American caregivers. These reasons for low service use support what has already been presented in the literature. In order to better serve this population, services must be affordable and available at times which are most needed by caregivers.

A finding somewhat inconsistent with previous research was the similar experience of emotional strain among all racial and ethnic groups. This finding raises questions about whether caregiver strain is in fact a predictor of formal service use, as suggested by our conceptual framework. If so, why do we see lower levels of formal service use among Asian/Native Hawaiian/Pacific Islander and Latina caregivers without also seeing differential strain among these caregivers? One possible explanation for this finding may be that those caregivers who experience cultural and language barriers to formal service use turn to informal support networks for assistance. These informal social networks are likely to have similar effects of reducing emotional strain on the caregiver. Another possible explanation, could be that a single-item measure of emotional strain may not be the best instrument to capture such a complex variable, leading us to caution the validity of its use.

Caregivers in all race and ethnicity categories tended to perceive themselves as making a contribution to their families and viewed the caregiving situation as one that included the whole family unit. Conflict or hardship in the family was rarely attributed to the caregiving situation. This may indicate that regardless of race or ethnicity, caregivers may turn to family members for assistance first. As previous research indicates, family networks of minority caregivers may be larger, thus providing more informal assistance before turning to formal service providers.

A one-size-fits-all approach to caregiver services is not likely to meet the needs of minority elders, and may in fact inhibit service use (Damskey, 2000). In developing interventions for ethnic minority elders and their caregivers, it is necessary to implement culturally sensitive interventions that incorporate caregivers' values and beliefs. Gallagher-Thompson et al. (2003) have suggested that the following factors are important when designing interventions for culturally diverse populations: (1) match the cultural background of the group and the intervention, (2) know what is relevant and sensitive to a group, (3) use culturally appropriate methods of communication, (4) use group members to help with implementation of an intervention, and (5) recognize that the effectiveness of an intervention is in part determined by its acceptance by key community leaders and other important individuals in the community.

When services are equally accessible and designed to be culturally sensitive, the decision to utilize formal services may be attributed less to predisposing variables such as race or cultural beliefs regarding health and service use, and more to enabling variables such as barriers to service use, or other variables which may or may not be defined differentially by race or ethnicity. Perhaps instead of using race as a proxy for understanding ethnic and cultural differences in caregiving, future research should include variables that allow for understanding the sociocultural characteristics of racial and ethnic minorities, including caregivers' own perceptions of the caregiving process. This will in turn provide more explanatory power for outcome measures and lead to more effectively designed research, practice, and educational programs.

CONCLUSION

The current article describes the family caregiving experience and formal service use among a statewide random sample of caregivers in California. The sample, the first of its kind, is relatively representative of the state, which has the largest and most diverse older adult population of any state within the U.S. The major findings presented here suggest that in order to help support family caregivers in their role, it is important to understand their needs for formal and informal support not only within the context of race and ethnicity, but within the broader socioeconomic and cultural contexts in which race and ethnicity exist.

Results from this study underscore the importance of the development of culturally competent caregiver services, especially when working with ethnically and culturally diverse clients. As reported by our respondents, culturally competent programming appears to be lacking or inadequate. Specifically, the current patterns of service utilization by Asian/Native Hawaiian/Pacific Islander and Latina caregivers are especially problematic. These two groups, when compared to White and African Americans, were significantly less likely to use formal caregiver services. They were also more likely to report a language barrier as the reason for not using services. A large proportion of Asian/Native Hawaiian/Pacific Islander and Latino Americans in the United States is foreign-born and speak a language other than English as a first language. In order to overcome existing service barriers faced by immigrant caregivers, service providers should strive to assure adequate linguistically appropriate service access and use for populations with limited English proficiency (LEP).

The significant differences in service utilization of White and African American caregivers compared with Asian/Native Hawaiian/Pacific Islander and Latina American caregivers also suggest that service use may be driven by a number of factors that interact with ethnicity. These factors, such as level of acculturation, language barriers, and living arrangements, to name a few, are important to consider for future research as well as in the development of public policy, programs, or educational curricula.

There were strengths and limitations worth noting in this study. The strength of the random sample provides us with a representative cross-section of caregivers in the state that allows us to examine patterns of service across several ethnicities in addition to White and African American. The limitations include the descriptive and therefore nontheoretical approach to studying racial and ethnic differences among caregivers, the underrepresentation of Asian caregivers, and finally, the somewhat limited measures of caregiver strain and well-being.

Future research is necessary to further understand the service spectrum needed to serve all caregivers and to continue to explore cultural values related to the caregiving experience and their implications for social work practice and education. Perhaps it is time to move beyond the behavioral model of medical service utilization and search for a newer model to explain service need and use, including informal as well as other types of community services. Qualitative approaches toward learning more about the role of cultural values in utilizing formal and informal services may be particularly helpful in comparing, and thus further understanding the caregiving process among various racial/ethnic groups. With this further understanding, social work educators will be better able to integrate these findings into curricula that emphasize cultural sensitivity, and social work practitioners will be better prepared to implement more sensitive services. Knowledge of the caregiving experience of an increasingly racially and ethnically diverse population will serve to clarify and enrich the picture for policy development and program implementation, while encompassing the variety of caregiver needs and situations.

REFERENCES

Ajrouch, K. J., Antonucci, T. C., & Janevic, M. R. (2001). Social networks among Blacks and Whites: The interaction between race and age. *Journal of Gerontology: Social Sciences, 56B*(2), S112-S118.

Andersen, R. M. (1995). Revisiting the behavioral model and access to medical care: Does it matter? *Journal of Health and Social Behavior, 36*(1), 1-10.

Andersen, R. M., & Newman, J. F. (1973). Societal and individual determinants of medical care utilization in the United States. *Milbank Memorial Fund Quarterly Journal, 51*, 95-124.

Aranda, M. P., & Knight, B. G. (1997). The influences of ethnicity and culture on the caregiver stress and coping process: A sociocultural review and analysis. *The Gerontologist, 37*, 342-357.

Bengtson, V., Rosenthal, C., & Burton, L. (1996). Paradoxes of families and aging. In R. Binstock & L. George (Eds.), *Handbook of Aging and the Social Sciences* (4th ed., pp. 254-282). New York: Academic Press.

Calsyn, R. J., & Winter, J. P. (2000). Predicting different types of service use by the elderly: The strength of the behavioral model and the value of interaction terms. *The Journal of Applied Gerontology, 19*(3), 284-303.

Census Bureau, U. S. (2000). Projections of the total resident population by 5-year age groups, race, and Hispanic origin with special age categories. U.S. Census website. Retrieved April 15, 2003, 2003, from the World Wide Web: www.census.gov/population/projections/nation/summary/np-t4-a.txt

Connell, C. M., & Gibson, G. D. (1997). Racial, ethnic, and cultural differences in dementia caregiving: Review and analysis. *The Gerontologist, 37*(3), 355-364.

Damskey, M. (2000). Views and visions: Moving toward culturally competent practice. In S. Alemán, T. Fitzpatrick, T. V. Tran, & E. W. Gonzalez (Eds.), *Therapeutic Interventions with Ethnic Elders: Health and Social Issues* (pp. 195-208). New York: The Haworth Press, Inc.

Dilworth-Anderson, P. (1995). *Cultural Justification Caregiving Scale* (unpublished measure).

Dilworth-Anderson, P., Williams, I. C., & Gibson, B. E. (2002). Issues of race, ethnicity, and culture in caregiving research: A 20-year review (1980-2000). *The Gerontologist, 42*(2), 237-272.

Dunlop, D. D., Manheim, L. M., Song, J., & Chang, R. W. (2002). Gender and ethnic/racial disparities in health care utilization among older adults. *Journal of Gerontology: Social Sciences, 57B*(3), S221-S235.

Gallagher-Thompson, D., Arean, P., Coon, D., Menendez, A., Takagi, K., Haley, W., Arguelles, T., Rubert, M., Lowenstein, D., & Szapocznik, J. (2000). Development and implementation of intervention strategies for culturally diverse caregiving populations. In R. Schulz (Ed.), *Handbook on Dementia Caregiving* (pp. 151-185). New York: Springer.

Gallagher-Thompson, D., Hargrave, R., Hinton, L., Arean, P., Iwamasa, G., & Zeiss, L. M. (2003). Interventions for a multicultural society. In D. Coon, D. Gallagher-Thompson, & L. W. Thompson (Eds.), *Innovative Interventions to Reduce Dementia Caregiver Distress* (pp. 50-73). New York: Springer.

General Accounting Office, U.S. (1995). *Long-Term Care: Current Issues and Future Directions*. Washington, DC: (GAO/HEHS-95-109).

Janevic, M. R., & Connell, C. M. (2001). Racial, ethnic, and cultural differences in the dementia caregiving experience: Recent findings. *The Gerontologist, 41*(3), 334-347.

Liu, K., & Manton, K. G. (1994). Changes in Home Care Use by Disabled Elderly Persons: 1982-1989 (Report for Congress, No. 94-398EPW). Washington, DC: U.S. Congressional Research Service.

Liu, K., Manton, K. G., & Aragon, C. (2000). *Changes in Home Care Use by Older People with Disabilities: 1982-1994*. Washington DC: AARP Public Policy Institute.

Mui, A. C., Choi, N. G., & Monk, A. (1998). *Long-Term Care and Ethnicity*. Westport, CT: Auburn House.

National Alliance for Caregiving and American Association of Retired Persons (1997). *Family Caregiving in the U.S.: Findings from a National Survey*. Washington, DC.

Navaie-Waliser, M., Feldman, P., Gould, D. A., Levine, C., Kuerbis, A. N., & Donelan, K. (2001). The experiences and challenges of informal caregivers: Common themes and differences among Whites, Blacks, and Hispanics. *The Gerontologist, 41*(6), 733-741.

Scharlach, A., & Greenlee, J. (2001). Caregivers' characteristics and needs. In A. Scharlach, T. Dal Santo, J. Greenlee, S. Whittier, D. Coon, K. Kietzman, K. Mills-Dick, P. Fox, & J. Aaker, *Family Caregivers In California: Needs, Interventions and Model Program*. Berkeley, CA: Center for the Advanced Study of Aging Services, University of California at Berkeley.

Scharlach, A., Sirotnik, B., Bockman, S., Neiman, M., Ruiz, C., & Dal Santo, T. (2003). *A Profile of Family Caregivers: Results of the California Statewide Survey of Caregivers*. Berkeley, CA: University of California Center for the Advanced Study of Aging Services.

Tennstedt, S., & Chang, B.-H. (1998). The relative contribution of ethnicity versus socioeconomic status in explaining differences in disability and receipt of informal care. *Journal of Gerontology: Social Sciences, 53B*(2), S61-S70.

Toseland, R. W., McCallion, P., Gerber, T., & Banks, S. (2002). Predictors of health and human services use by persons with dementia and their family caregivers. *Social Science & Medicine, 55*(7), 1255-1266.

White-Means, S. I., & Thornton, M. C. (1996). Well-being among caregivers of indigent Black elderly. *Journal of Comparative Family Studies, 27*(1), 109-128.

Yeatts, D. E., Crow, T., & Folts, E. (1992). Service use among low-income minority elderly: Strategies for overcoming barriers. *The Gerontologist, 32*(1), 24-32.

APPENDIX

Selected Items from California Caregiver Survey Instrument

Caregiver Characteristics

- Gender
- Age
- Race/Ethnicity
- Relationship to CR
- Education level
- Income
- Marital status
- Children under age 18 living in the home

Service Utilization

"Have you received . . ."

- Information about community services for yourself or your (care-receiver relationship)?
- Help getting or using community services?
- Professional counseling?
- Information about your legal rights and obligations as a care provider?
- If respondent answered yes to any of the above, he or she was asked whether they received the service from family, friends, an agency, or other source.

Service Barriers

"Reasons you have not received more outside help caring for your (care-receiver relationship)"

- Already have all the help you need.
- Your (relationship) does not want it.
- Service quality is poor.
- Service providers don't speak your language.
- Transportation is not available.

Strain and Coping

On a scale from 1 to 5,

- How much of a financial hardship would you say that caring for your (relationship) is for you?
- How much of a physical strain would you say that caring for your (relationship) is for you?
- How emotionally stressful would you say that caring for your (relationship) is for you?

How much has this situation . . .

- Brought your family closer together?
- Created conflict or disagreements in your family?
- Been a hardship for your family?

How often do you usually . . .

- Attend religious services, meetings, and/or activities?
- Pray or meditate on your own?

PART II

RACE

The Ethics
of Medical Decision-Making
with Japanese-American Elders in Hawaii:
Signing Informed Consent Documents
Without Understanding Them

Morris Saldov

Hisako Kakai

SUMMARY. This study reports observations by oncology nurses, doctors, social workers and administrators at Queen's Medical Center

Morris Saldov, MSW, PhD, School of Social Work, is Associate Professor of Social Work, Monmouth University. Hisako Kakai, PhD, is affiliated with the School of International Politics, Economics, and Business at Aoyama Gakuin University.

This paper is based upon a study that was completed with the assistance of a joint grant from the Social Welfare Education Research Unit, School of Social Work, University of Hawaii and the Queen's Medical Center (QMC) Research Foundation in Honolulu.

[Haworth co-indexing entry note]: "The Ethics of Medical Decision-Making with Japanese-American Elders in Hawaii: Signing Informed Consent Documents Without Understanding Them." Saldov, Morris, and Hisako Kakai. Co-published simultaneously in *Journal of Human Behavior in the Social Environment* (The Haworth Social Work Practice Press, an imprint of The Haworth Press, Inc.) Vol. 10, No. 1, 2004, pp. 113-130; and: *Diversity and Aging in the Social Environment* (eds: Sherry M. Cummings, and Colleen Galambos) The Haworth Social Work Practice Press, an imprint of The Haworth Press, Inc., 2004, pp. 113-130. Single or multiple copies of this article are available for a fee from The Haworth Document Delivery Service [1-800-HAWORTH, 9:00 a.m. - 5:00 p.m. (EST). E-mail address: docdelivery@haworthpress.com].

(QMC) in Honolulu (N = 50), concerning cultural, religious and institutional factors influencing mentally competent Japanese-American elders signing medical informed consent (IC) documents without understanding them. Sixty-eight percent of respondents reported having observed elderly Japanese-Americans signing IC documents without understanding them. Explanatory concepts of *enryo* (refraining from imposing one's own interest or desire), *oyakoko* (filial piety), *ishin-denshin* (silent communication) and *obasute* (a traditional practice of sacrificing oneself to avoid being a burden to others), in addition to other cultural concepts are discussed for their possible contribution to "signing without understanding." Suggestions are made for further research to include elders and their family members to explore the perceptions of IC. The study concludes with recommendations for improvements to the laws, policies, programs and procedures governing the IC process in order to achieve a better fit with the cultural, ethnic and religious characteristics of Japanese-American elderly patients in America. *[Article copies available for a fee from The Haworth Document Delivery Service: 1-800-HAWORTH. E-mail address: <docdelivery@haworthpress.com> Website: <http://www.HaworthPress.com>* © *2004 by The Haworth Press, Inc. All rights reserved.]*

KEYWORDS. Ethics, informed, consent, Japanese-American elders

INTRODUCTION

According to the Self-Determination Act (1991), informed consent in America requires that individual patients be active participants in their own medical decision-making irrespective of ethno-cultural or religious differences. The concept of self in America is an individual one. In Japanese and other Asian cultures the concept of self is enmeshed in family and community. The conflict between legal obligations to conform to the Self-Determination Act and the ethical requirements of cultural competency are highlighted in this study. Individual patients signing informed consent documents without understanding them is a violation of the Act. Even though doctors may adhere to the law, by not involving family or significant members of the Japanese community, they may be in breach of their own code of ethics requiring that cultural competency be applied to the IC procedure.

The study from which this paper is drawn was initially developed in response to an observation by the head of the Social Work Department at QMC that a large number of Japanese-American elderly being treated for cancer were having a problem participating in the IC procedure. Several problems were identified including: delays in obtaining consent resulting in extended length of stays (LOS) and possible time elapsing before treatments were rendered; confusion and related stress on the patient and their families when respective roles in decision-making were unclear; patients signing consents without truly understanding them. An earlier study (Saldov, Kakai, McLaughlin, & Thomas, 1998) examined the problems associated with delays in obtaining consent. This paper examines a variety of factors that may have contributed to Japanese- American elderly patients signing IC documents without understanding them. To investigate this observation further, oncology health care staff including doctors, nurses, social workers, and program managers were asked to relate their experiences with Japanese-American elderly patients.

The ethics of IC are both controversial and problematic. While there is both an ethical and legal obligation as part of the IC procedure to educate and inform individual patients of their diagnosis and treatment options, it is also expected that health care workers will respect their cultural and religious preferences. Patients who prefer to exercise a cultural or religious value of non-participation or deferral of decision-making may choose to sign IC documents without understanding them. When health care workers respect cultural or religious values and beliefs dictating the deferral of medical decision-making to someone else, their response may be viewed as a sign of compliance with the requirements for cultural competency in their professional codes of ethics. However, this cultural responsiveness can sometimes come into conflict with the legal and ethical requirements for disclosing a diagnosis and obtaining IC.

This study was designed to report and analyze the QMC staff's observations of factors influencing Japanese-American elderly patients signing IC documents without understanding them. Results of this exploratory descriptive study are expected to lead to further research which can help identify procedures that may achieve a better fit between the IC procedure and the Japanese-American elders' cultural and religious practices and beliefs.

THEORETICAL FRAMEWORK: PERSON-ENVIRONMENT CONGRUENCE MODEL

Person-Environment Congruence Theory provides a common-sense model for policymakers, managers, and professionals to achieve a better fit between the health environments they create and the people they purport to serve (Kahana, 1982). A congruence model may supply a systematic set of guidelines sought by health care professionals to accomplish such a match when working with the Japanese-American elderly in Hawaii. There is a need to match the health services environment to background characteristics of culture and religion variables in particular. Within the congruence model, whenever there is a mismatch between the individual's needs and his or her life situation due to either change in environment like hospitalization, or a change in needs or abilities, adaptive strategies are required to improve the fit between person and environment. Adaptive strategies are needed, particularly in the field of ethnogerontological oncology, to reduce the mismatch either by changing behavior or by altering the environment (Garcia & Lee, 1988). Depending on the "goodness of fit" of these adaptive strategies, well-being or lack of it may result.

Individuals strive within a formal service structure and informal systems of social support networks to meet all of their biopsychosocial requirements. The congruence between consumers of health care and their social support networks and formal services determines the goodness of fit. Getzinger (1993) has suggested that there is a need to examine the extent of congruence between the American health care system applying the IC procedure and the characteristics of different cultural groups being served.

How well do health care services match the requirements of Japanese-American elderly patients and their families when it comes to obtaining IC? The congruence question asks if the systems of support services are matched with the varying needs of diverse cultural and religious groups.

HAWAII'S ETHNIC ELDER MINORITIES

In 1990, the Japanese population over 60 years old represented nearly half (47%) of the six major elderly groups in Hawaii (see Table 1). While Japanese, Filipino, Chinese, Hawaiian and Korean elderly are more populous in Hawaii and California, they represent less than 1% of the senior population of the U.S. (Census, CP-3-5, 1990).

Japanese make up the largest group of elderly health care consumers in Hawaii. Tamura (1994) has noted that the Issei (first generation) and to a lesser extent the Nissei (second generation-Hawaii born) have tended to retain traditional values like *enryo* which inclines the elders to defer to the authority of persons with greater power distance from them.

TABLE 1. Major Ethnic Elderly Groups in Hawaii (age 60 and Over in 1990)

Chinese	Filipino	Hawaiian	Japanese	Korean	White	Total
15,129	24,477	12,261	66,940	3,655	18,748	141,210
10.7%	17.3%	8.7%	47.4%	2.6%	13.3%	100%

Source: 1990 Census of Population: General Population Characteristics, Hawaii, CP 1-13. U.S. Census 2000 does not provide the Hawaii data by age and race.

The tendency to act in ways promoting harmony and interdependent relations or *amae* (Doi, 1962) among traditional Japanese may also incline the Japanese-American elderly towards signing consents without understanding them. Hawaii's predominance of Japanese-American elderly presents a unique opportunity to study ethical issues as they relate to cultural and religious factors in medical decision-making.

JAPANESE CULTURAL VALUES AND HEALTH CARE

Dependency on family members (*amae*), deference to persons in authority (*enryo*) for caregiving in old age, and protection by doctors and family from disclosure to the elders of serious illnesses (*yasurakani*), may be expected values in traditional Japanese culture. Added to these traditional values are silent communication styles (*ishin-denshin*), which further prevent disclosure and discussion of serious illnesses (see Glossary of Terms). Many Japanese-Americans expect their families to play a significant role in their caregiving (*oyakoko*) (Long & Long, 1982; Ohnuki-Tierney, 1984). This role may include taking over critical medical decisions even though the patient signs IC documents without being informed about or understanding the diagnosis, prognosis, or alternative treatment options. According to Hattori et al. (1991), some of the cultural factors which may lead to the family taking this role in traditional Japanese culture include (a) priority of collective family interests over those of individuals, (b) preservation of harmony, (c) responsibility for care of the elderly by the family (*oyakoko*), (d) psychology of dependency of the patient on the family (*amae*) that validates collectivistic or interdependent ways of relating with family members and confidantes, and (e) a family's desire to let their loved one "die in peace" (*yasurakani*), without the patient experiencing the agony of knowing the true diagnosis. In Japan, oncologists have often withheld a diagnosis of cancer from their patients for this reason, preferring instead to share medical information with family members (Tanida, 1994).

During the course of a patient's terminal illness the traditional role of physicians and family members is to shield the truth from the patient as much as possible so that she or he does not learn of the negative prognosis (Long & Long, 1982). If the patient is an elderly parent, it may be particularly important not to communicate a diagnosis of terminal illness. The traditional expectation in Japanese culture that the elderly will be looked after by family or the doctors (*oyakoko*), may otherwise be thwarted. The absence of *oyakoko* can result in feelings of shame due to the elder perceiving a lack of caregiving. Many Japanese in America will not express the expectation that filial obligation be observed, being reluctant to ask others on whom they depend (*amae*) to take care of them, fearing that they may be disappointed by their family members' lack of a response. With this fear, elders may be likely to refrain from imposing themselves on others (*enryo*), thereby reinforcing a kind of social deference which allows for acceptance of unsolicited caring behavior from others (Tamura, 1994).

The concept of *enryo* has also been interpreted as "refraining from expressing disagreement with whatever appears to be the majority's opinion" (Lebra, 1976, p. 29). Traditional Japanese-American elders who think this way may be expected to adopt a passive role when it comes to potentially contentious medical decision-making and therefore sign IC documents without understanding them. Owing to this traditional value of *enryo*, family members may be further discouraged from disclosing the true diagnosis of a serious illness to a Japanese elder.

The patient's expected role has been to leave physicians and family members to deal with their illness, even if the patient finds out about his or her condition (Long & Long, 1982). Patients signing IC documents under these circumstances may prefer not to be informed by doctors and family members, thereby allowing them to "die in peace" (*yasurakani*), comforted in the knowledge that family members and physicians are looking after their best interests (*oyakoko*) (Ohnuki-Tierney, 1984).

If patients sign out of deference to doctors or an eldest son, but do not know of their condition, they may be unable to share feelings with family members or professional caregivers. This lack of communication can lead to a lonely process of dying (*sabishii shi*) (Ohnuki-Tierney, 1984). However, persons diagnosed with a terminal illness in Japan may not suffer *sabishii shi* when there is no discussion of their illness. Family members may be giving support to patients by using the traditional practice of silent communication (*ishin-denshin*), in which true meanings are often exchanged non-verbally (Marsella, 1993). *Ishin-denshin* communicates heartfelt understanding without saying words. This form of non-verbal communication is neither denial of an illness by the patient or family members nor avoidance through lack of discussion. Rather, it is a traditional Japanese practice using indirect forms of communication aimed at maintaining social awareness and harmonious relationships.

Elders may sometimes hesitate to obtain medical treatment due to worries about imposing monetary, psychological, or physical stresses on family members. Honoring patients' preference not to be told their diagnosis, prognosis or treatment options may assist them in avoiding feelings that they are a burden to anyone. Family members and doctors knowing this preference may be inclined to withhold information to prevent the elders from experiencing these burdensome feelings. To avoid being a burden is a strong traditional belief in Japanese culture. In ancient Japan, avoidance of being a burden was institutionalized as the practice of *obasute*, whereby Japanese elders frequently sacrificed their lives when their villages were short of resources (Takamura, 1991).

Takamura found that Japanese men in Hawaii who were 85 years of age and older had almost three times the suicide rates of their white male counterparts. This difference was accounted for by suggesting that some Japanese men continue to support the principles inherent in the practice of *obasute*. In contrast to Japanese females, who have been perceived to be more passive and dependent,[1] Japanese males have been viewed as being more aggressive and independent. It has been suggested that the high rates of suicide by elderly Japanese-American males in Hawaii is representative of the need to exercise control over their lives and to avoid being seen as weak and dependent, particularly when the elder identifies himself as having been invincible like a Samurai warrior. In this case the honorable way out of becoming a burden is to commit suicide.

Japanese elderly following *obasute* may also seek to sacrifice themselves because of the belief that their continued existence could jeopardize their children's or their grandchildren's marriage chances. If it becomes widely known that a family member is afflicted with a serious illness like cancer, that knowledge may be seen as limiting the marriageability of offspring owing to ideas about cancer's inheritability.

JAPANESE RELIGIOUS BELIEFS

Religion has played an important role in medical decision-making in modern Japan (Ohnuki-Tierney, 1984). Japanese perceptions of illness may not only be influenced by cultural values but also by religious beliefs. Long and Long (1982) have pointed to the influences of Shintoism, which promote the belief that poor health is the consequence of a socially polluted spirit (*kegare*). Japanese believing in *kegare* may experience strong social stigma when suffering from a serious disease such as cancer. They will not want to discuss such an illness for fear of spiritually contaminating others. Therefore, discussion of terminal diseases may be avoided (Long & Long, 1982; Ohnuki-Tierney, 1984).

In ancient Japan the concept of "*kotodama*" embodied the belief that a word had its own soul. "*Koto*" means "word" and "*dama*" refers to the "soul" (Itasaka, 1971). Undesirable events were believed to happen once someone actually spoke about a possible negative occurrence. Talking about such things as death or a serious illness is discouraged even in modern Japan. Therefore, non-disclosure by oncologists and family members in Japan may not only derive from paternalistic medical practices or emphasis on cultural values of harmony (*enryo*) and consensus (*amae*) in decision-making (Feldman, 1985), but it may also originate from beliefs in *kegare* or *kotodama*.

If there are strong beliefs in avoiding discussion of their illness and in seeking recovery through prayer, Japanese elderly's participation in medical decision-making may also be highly unlikely. Traditional Japanese elders who subscribe to Taoist and Buddhist perceptions of illness often believe that suffering is an essential part of life. Stoic endurance of illness (*gaman*), under Taoism and Buddhism, becomes a highly valued practice (Reynolds & Kicfer, 1977; Marsella, 1993). Many Japanese elderly subscribe to the fatalism and harmony of Buddhist philosophy which, in contrast to the Western values of controlling nature, embraces the idea of living harmoniously with their natural environment.

Many of the values and religious beliefs discussed here, those of *enryo, amae, kotodama, kegare, obasute, yasurakani, gaman, ishin-den-shin, oyakoko, sabishii shi*, point to the possibility that traditional Japanese elders may be more likely to sign IC documents without understanding them. Dependency on family members, deference to persons in authority for caregiving in old age, and protection by doctors from disclosure to the elders of serious illnesses are strongly held values in traditional Japanese culture.

CONDITIONS FOR INFORMED CONSENT

The doctrine of IC grew out of the 1960s social movement for consumers' rights in the U.S. When the struggle extended to the health care field, it resulted in a clash between medical paternalism and patient autonomy (Edge & Groves, 1994). This conflict was somewhat settled by the adoption of the Patients' Bill of Rights (1973), the implementation of self-determination clauses in the Health Professions' Codes of Ethics and the passage of the Patient Self-Determination Act (1990).

It is assumed that in the U.S., patients will exercise their right as knowledgeable participants to manage their own health care. The medical IC procedure is used to ensure that the patient has the right to needed information to direct his or her care. For doctors, adherence to the policy of IC is both an ethical and a legal obligation. Physicians must disclose a diagnosis to their patients, outline the options for treatment, and make recommendations in order to obtain voluntary consent, before giving medical treatment (Edge & Groves 1994). The IC procedure entails: (a) disclosure–sharing of diagnosis by physician to patient; (b) understanding–disclosure of information regarding treatment in a form that is understandable to the patient; (c) free will–patient is not coerced or manipulated to make a decision; (d) competence–patient is able to exhibit sound judgement; and (e) consent–patient authorizes the medical intervention. Medical decision-making by a patient can only be deferred to someone else when she or he is mentally incompetent or has exercised a Durable Power of Attorney (DPOA) for health care.

Health care professionals in the U.S. may be challenged, however, when cultural conflicts lead medical decision-making away from the personal autonomy of the patient towards collectivist decision-making. When seeking consent from a traditional Japanese-American elder, the patient's preference may be to have the diagnosis withheld, leaving decisions about medical care to the doctor, family members, or both. Even though the elders may sign, decisions about treatment are left up to their caregivers.

Mentally competent traditional Japanese-American elderly may prefer to defer their medical decision-making either to their eldest son, or another family member, their doctor, or both. They may not even want to know their diagnosis, prognosis or options for treatment. Under these conditions, how is IC possible, given the legal requirement for understanding their medical circumstances in order to give consent?

The ethics of IC in large part agree with the legal requirements for self-determination, which are consistently found in the Codes of Ethics of all the Health Professions. The ethical-legal conflict arises, however, when the professional obligation to apply skills for culturally competent practice dictates that patients be able to sign IC documents without understanding them if that is their preference. The Patient Self-Determination Act (1990) requires that medical staff obtain IC from mentally competent patients. The ethical obligation to educate patients and involve them in medical decision-making complicates the IC conundrum, as this principle may conflict with the additional ethical requirement to respect the cultural characteristics and preferences of clients who may not want to know their diagnosis or participate in their treatment. The right to self-determination includes choosing not to be informed of a diagnosis and not to be involved in the medical decision-making. When there is a cultural preference not to disclose an illness or to include the patient in the IC process, the family and the physician, using "therapeutic privilege," may keep the diagnosis from the patient (Edge & Groves, 1994).

In the case of a traditional Japanese-American elder who wishes neither to be informed nor to give IC, professional and cultural competence in medical practice demands that these preferences be respected. Therefore, signing IC documents without understanding them may not be a problem of language or other barriers to executing the procedure. Rather, signing without understanding may well be executing a cultural preference for self-determination through deferral of decision-making to others. The doctor's decision to invoke therapeutic privilege is based upon his or her judgement that the effects of disclosure would be harmful to the patient. In Hawaii where there is a large population of Japanese-American elders, cultural and religious differences have challenged the health care system to be adaptive to preferences varying from mainstream Western medical practices.

RESEARCH METHODS

A convenience sample of 50 was drawn from a population of 161 health care staff (31% response rate), including three medical and radiation oncologists, 27 nurses, three program managers, and 17 social workers. Reasons cited by staff at the hospital for the low response rate include: reduced priority given to research in times of staff shortages; and the sensitive nature of the research such as the risks of exposing illegal or unethical practices when seeking informed consent for treatment. Forty-six respondents were females (see Table 2).

TABLE 2. Demographic Characteristics of 50 Participants

Variables	Categories	Frequency	Percent
Gender	Female	46	92%
Ethnicity	Caucasian	22	44%
	Japanese	9	18%
	Mixed	7	14%
	Filipino	3	6%
	Chinese	2	4%
	Hispanic	1	2%
	missing case	6	12%
Professions	MDs	3	6%
	Nurses	27	54%
	Program mgrs	3	6%
	Social workers	17	34%
Length of experience	Less than 6 yrs	23	46%
	6 years or more	27	54%

A majority of the participants were Caucasian (22 out of 50), followed by Japanese (9), mixed race (7), Filipino (3), Chinese (2), and Hispanic (1), with six missing cases. There were six cases where ethnic identity was not reported. More than half of the respondents (27) had worked in health care settings for six years or more.

Questions in the survey, developed from the literature review on Japanese culture, were tested for content validity through consultations with key informants both from academic and health care practice settings (see Appendix). Participation on the study team by the Manager of the Social Work Department at QMC helped researchers to understand the hospital context for the study. Involvement by an overseas student from Japan specializing in cross-cultural studies enhanced the literature review and understanding of key concepts in Japanese culture. A colloquium was held at the University of Hawaii, School of Social Work, to help clarify research objectives and methodology. Health care, legal, and educational staff participated in a focus group to aid in the refinement of the survey questions. Questionnaires were pilot tested at two other Honolulu hospitals (Kuakini Medical Center and St. Francis Hospital), which also served Japanese-American elderly oncology patients. A letter was sent by the Manager of the Social Work Department to the other Departmental Managers explaining the rationale and auspices of the research to encourage participation in the study. Questionnaires were distributed to the various departments and collected at departmental drop points. Two follow-up reminder letters were delivered to departments to encourage a higher response rate. Questionnaires took from 10-20 minutes to complete.

FINDINGS

A majority of participants (34 out of 50) reported that they had observed what they believed to be cases of Japanese-American elderly oncology patients signing IC documents without understanding them (see Table 3).

Four respondents reported that they had not observed Japanese-American elderly patients sign IC documents without understanding them, while the remainder (11) said that they were unsure. There was no opportunity to cross-validate these findings as neither the elders nor their family members participated in this study. For those who reported differences across age groups, almost all (11 out of 12) observed more Japanese-American elderly patients who were 80 years or older signing without understanding.

Of those participants who reported that they had observed patients sign the documents without understanding them, 14 out of 30 thought it was because they were deferring decision-making to oncologists. Many Japanese-American elderly patients trust and respect the oncologists for their expert knowledge to do what is best for them. These elders, especially female patients, do not want to challenge the authority of the oncologist by being assertive, inquisitive or disagreeable (*enryo* and *amae*). They may also fear the doctor's loss of face over their non-compliance with treatment. Japanese culture has always emphasized respecting authority through acceptance of the status quo social power distribution. Therefore, Japanese-American elders with strong traditional values of power distance will readily comply with doctors' treatment orders.

TABLE 3. Frequency of Reported Cases of Signing Without Understanding

Signing I.C. documents without understanding	Frequency	Percent
Yes	34	68%
No	4	8%
Not sure	11	22%
Missing case	1	2%
Total	50	100%

The role of family members is reflected in the observations of participants in the study. For example, it was reported that family members, acting as translators, tended to keep controversial information from patients (*amae* and *yasurakani*). The absence of family members at the time of obtaining consent departs from traditional family obligations (*oyakoko*). This sometimes draws attention to the shame of family members who are not living up to their filial obligations of looking after their elders (*amae* and *oyakoko*), perhaps causing loneliness, fear, confusion and isolation (*sabishii shi*) at a critical time when needed to support their elders. From a Western point of view, *oyakoko* (filial piety) may interfere with the patient's right to self-determination but presents no such conflict in traditional Japanese culture. Elders who expect their children to look after them may not want to know about their diagnosis, prognosis or treatment, preferring to leave medical decisions to family members. While linguistic and cultural communication barriers were not listed as reasons why patients signed without understanding, they may represent another set of factors contributing to deferral of medical decision-making. The barriers to communication might not be limited to language but also to Japanese-American elderly patients' lack of knowledge about modern diagnostic methods and treatment options. The frequent use of medical jargon in discussing diagnosis and treatment also presents problems in communicating with all patients and may therefore not be unique to the Japanese-American elderly. Participants noted that oncologists do not spend sufficient time in explaining the diagnosis, treatment options, and prognoses to Japanese-American elderly patients, thereby cutting short the IC procedure. These short cuts may be due to communication barriers or paying attention to cultural sensitivities. Pressure placed on the elders by family members who are protective, respect by the elder for power distance of the oncologist, and the time limitations on treatment imposed by the Diagnosis Related Groups (DRG) system of Medicare/Medicaid payment, may also help to explain why elders signed IC forms without understanding them. These institutional factors were not fully explored by respondents in their answers given.

To help explain the observation by health care workers that Japanese-American elderly frequently signed IC documents without understanding them, further research needs to be undertaken examining the complex set of relationships between institutional, cultural, and religious factors influencing medical decision-making.

LIMITATIONS OF THE STUDY

While these results may suggest trends in explaining why Japanese-American elders at QMC signed IC documents without understanding them, cautious interpretation is warranted by the small sample size of staff and the lack of involvement in the study by elders and their family members. Participation by 50 staff members in a major hospital setting is too small to generate much analysis or obtain statistical significance from the data. Additionally, in a number of cases there were missing data reducing the sample size even further. Also, the predominantly Caucasian composition of the sample may have contributed to less awareness of cultural factors influencing participation in medical decision-making by Japanese-American elderly and their family members. The absence of input from the population under study, that is, the Japanese-American elderly patients and their family members in Hawaii is problematic. Data on the elders and their families is needed to cross-validate the findings on the views of health care professionals. Findings from this exploratory study nevertheless suggest that more systematic research is needed to take into account the views of Japanese-American elders and their family members on the topic of IC.

IMPLICATIONS FOR POLICY AND PRACTICE

Although there appears to be a growing interest in cultural competency when executing the IC procedure,[2] to date no policy to guarantee a systematic approach to facilitating complex medical decision-making has been adopted as part of the U.S. health care agenda. The complexity of the consent procedure and the propensity in America towards patients' and consumers' rights, with its ever present threat of litigation, may point to a greater need to develop a more systematic approach to obtaining IC with culturally and religiously diverse populations. Health care practitioners working with traditional ethnic elderly will increasingly be required to demonstrate to the patients and their family members, to their own professions, and to the courts when necessary, that they have taken every reasonable step to ensure ethical practices when obtaining consent. Conflicts between traditional and modern, Eastern and Western values may be exposed when consent is sought from Japanese-American elders in the U.S. (Kitano & Daniels, 1995), particularly in Hawaii (Tamura, 1994). These populations become fertile groups for research to help develop a larger database to better inform the procedure for obtaining IC. In the case of Japanese and perhaps other Asian elderly in America, cultural and religious differences from Western modes of decision-making provide an opportunity and a challenge for health care professionals to develop an IC procedure congruent with these diverse backgrounds. Some additional steps, which would demonstrate a commitment to culturally competent practice in medical decision-making might include, from a policy and practice perspective, instituting a pre-admission clinic wherein social workers are called upon to assess patterns of decision-making by patients and their families. In a critical care situation social workers would be called in through emergency department or critical care wards to assess the individual patients and their family members' norms for medical decision-making. These patterns may be susceptible to cultural, religious, or ethnic norms, which need to be respected when implementing the informed consent procedure. Social workers' assessments can therefore play an important role in educating and cooperating with medical staff charged with taking informed consent from diverse elderly populations. Additionally, social workers can become more active on institutional ethics committees, review boards and risk management committees in hospitals to help raise the issues related to conflicts between legal and ethical obligations of the health professions as they relate to taking of medical informed consent. At a macro level, the health professions can join in an advocacy effort to reform the Self-Determination Act in order to broaden the concept of self to incorporate different cultural, religious, and ethnic constructions. Continuing to define the self as an individual, in the face of evidence that at least some patients prefer family participation or deferral to caregivers in medical decision-making, will continue to present health professionals with the difficult choice between having to act legally in conformity with the Act or ethically in compliance with cultural competency requirements of their codes of ethics. Establishing some congruence between laws and ethics will help to end this dilemma. Changing the Self-Determination Act to allow for deferral to family or significant others without having to be declared mentally incompetent or medically unable to participate in the IC procedure would go a long way towards achieving this congruence.

GLOSSARY OF JAPANESE TERMS

Amae–Psychological dependency encouraging collectivistic inter-relationships among family members.

Enryo–To hold back or refrain from imposing oneself on others.

Gaman–Buddhist belief in stoic endurance.

Ishin-denshin–To understand without saying words.

Kegare–Spiritual contamination.

Kotodama–Belief that words have their own soul, leading to the belief that undesirable events will happen once the words are spoken.

Obasute–The practice of elders imposing their own death as an honorable self-sacrifice when there is a shortage of resources.

Oyakoko–Filial piety (respect for parents)

Sabishii-Shi–A lonely process of dying.

Yasurakani–Allowing loved ones to "die in peace"; leads to the practice of withholding information from patients.

NOTES

1. The gender difference in responding to the sense of burden experienced by males inclines them towards taking their own lives, says Patty Demeroto, oncology social worker at Kuakini Medical Center. She has pointed out that males, who are often the breadwinners and have been accustomed to taking leadership roles, when afflicted with cancer, tend to see themselves as a burden to the family. Consequently, they may be inclined towards suicide as a means of relieving the family of any potential burdens.

2. A recent NIH call for research proposals to investigate cultural and ethnic sensitivities in obtaining IC for clinical research reveals a strategic research interest by the U.S. Government in this area (NIH RFA No. 97001, 1996). The American Society on Aging (ASA) Multicultural Aging Training and Networking Initiative is a further indication of the recent emphasis being given to education and research on culturally competent practice with the elderly (ASA, 1997).

REFERENCES

Census of Population (1990). Asian and Pacific islanders in the U.S. CP-3-5. Washington, DC: U.S. Government Printing Office.

Doi, T. (1962). "Amae": A key concept for understanding Japanese personality structure. In R.J. Smith & R.K. Beardsley (Eds.), *Japanese culture: Its development and characteristics*(pp. 132-139). Chicago: Aldine.

Edge, R.S., & Groves, J.R. (1994). *The ethics of health care: A guide for clinical practice.* Albany: Delmar Publishers Inc.

Feldman, E. (1985). Medical ethics the Japanese way. *Hastings Center Report, 15* (5), 21-24.

Garcia, H.B., & Lee, P.C.Y. (1988). Knowledge about cancer and use of health care services among Hispanic and Asian-American older adults. *Journal of Psychosocial Oncology, 16* (3/4), 157-177.

Getzinger, A. (1993). Informed consent and systems consultation: A description of the process and a prescription for change. *Family Systems Medicine, 11* (3), 235-245.

Hattori, H., Salzberg, S.M., Kiang, W.P. Fujimiya, T., Tejima, Y., & Furuno, J. (1991). The patient's right to information in Japan–legal rules and doctor's opinions. *Social Science and Medicine, 32* (9), 1007-1016.

Itasaka, G. (1971). Nihonjin no ronri kouzou [Japanese structure of logic]. Tokyo: Kodan-sha, Co., Ltd.

Kahana, E. (1982). A congruence model of person-environment interaction. In M.P. Lawton, P.G. Windley, & T.O. Byerts (Eds.), *Aging and the environment. Theoretical approaches* (pp. 97-121). New York: Springer.

Kitano, H., & Daniels, R. (1995). *Asian Americans: Emerging minorities* (2nd. ed.) Englewood Cliffs: Prentice-Hall.

Lebra, S.T. (1976). *Japanese patterns of behavior.* Honolulu: University of Hawaii Press.

Long, S.O., & Long, B.D. (1982). Curable cancers and fatal ulcers: Attitudes toward cancer in Japan. *Social Science and Medicine, 16,* 2101-2108.

Marsella, A.J. (1993). Counseling and psychotherapy with Japanese Americans: Cross-cultural considerations. *American Journal of Orthopsychiatry, 62*(2), 200-208.

Ohnuki-Tierney, E. (1984). *Illness and culture in contemporary Japan: An anthropological view.* Cambridge: Cambridge University Press.

Patient Self-Determination Act (1990). An act of congress passed as part of the Omnibus Budget Reconciliation Act (OBRA). Washington, DC: U.S. Government Printing Office.

Reynolds, D.K., & Kiefer, C.W. (1977). Cultural adaptability as an attribute of therapies: The case of Morita psychotherapy. *Culture, Medicine and Psychiatry, 1,* 395-412.

Saldov, M., Kakai, H., McLaughlin, L., & Thomas, A. (1998). Cultural barriers in oncology: Issues in obtaining medical informed consent from Japanese-American elders in Hawaii. *Journal of Cross-Cultural Gerontology, 13,* 265-279.

Takahashi, E. (1996). *Sei to shi no tonari awaseni* [Between life and death]. Tokyo: Kindaieiga-sha.

Takamura, J. C. (1991). Asian and Pacific Islander elderly. In N. Mokuau, (Ed.), *Handbook of social services for Asian and Pacific Islanders.* Westport CT: Greenwood Press.

Tamura, E.H. (1994). *Americanization, acculturation, and ethnic identity: The nisei generation in Hawaii.* Chicago, IL: University of Illinois Press.

Tanida, N. (1994). Japanese attitudes towards truth disclosure in cancer. *Scandinavian Journal of Social Medicine, 22*(1), 50-57.

APPENDIX

Questions About Signing IC Without Understanding

1. Have you ever experienced or heard of cases where a Japanese elderly patient did not fully understand the diagnosis, prognosis, and treatment options before signing the Medical IC?
2. How often would you estimate that a Japanese elderly patient signs Medical IC, when there is lack of understanding of the diagnosis, prognosis, and treatment options? (always, often, sometimes, rarely, not sure [please explain]).
3. Of the Japanese elderly oncology patients that you have worked with during the past year, roughly how many do you estimate signed Medical IC without fully understanding it?
4. What do you believe to be the major reason that Japanese elderly sign IC documents without understanding their diagnosis, prognosis, and treatment options?
5. From your recollection, have you noticed any difference in signing Medical IC without understanding when the patient is very old (80 and over), or relatively old (between 65-79 years old)?
6. Have you observed any gender differences in Japanese elderly signing Medical IC without understanding?
[If you have indicated a difference between males and females, please explain what you have noticed.]

Acculturation and Depressive Symptoms in Mexican American Couples

Margie Rodríguez Le Sage
Aloen Townsend

SUMMARY. Despite interest in examining the relationship between acculturation and depressive symptomatology among Latinos, limited attention has been given to these factors within the context of the Latino marital environment. The present study examines the role of acculturation in determining depressive symptoms among 173 married, Mexican American (MA) couples who participated in the 1992 Health and Retirement Survey, Wave I, while holding relevant variables (i.e., age, years of formal education, logged lower body difficulties, logged household income, logged household net worth, and logged household size) constant.

Margie Rodríguez Le Sage, LMSW, PhD, is Assistant Professor, School of Social Work, Michigan State University. Aloen Townsend, PhD, is Associate Professor, Mandel School of Applied Social Sciences, Case Western Reserve University.

Address correspondence to: Margie Rodríguez Le Sage, School of Social Work, Michigan State University, 254 Baker Hall, East Lansing, MI 48824 (E-mail: margie.rodriguezlesage@ssc.msu.edu).

This study is supported by the National Institute on Aging (Grant 1 RO1 AG17546).

This paper was presented in symposium, *Highlighting Interdependence in Mid Life and Late Life Married Couples*, A.L. Townsend and B. Miller (Chairs), at the 54th Annual Scientific Meeting of the American Gerontological Society of America, Chicago, November 2001.

[Haworth co-indexing entry note]: "Acculturation and Depressive Symptoms in Mexican American Couples." Le Sage, Margie Rodríguez, and Aloen Townsend. Co-published simultaneously in *Journal of Human Behavior in the Social Environment* (The Haworth Social Work Practice Press, an imprint of The Haworth Press, Inc.) Vol. 10, No. 1, 2004, pp. 131-154; and: *Diversity and Aging in the Social Environment* (eds: Sherry M. Cummings, and Colleen Galambos) The Haworth Social Work Practice Press, an imprint of The Haworth Press, Inc., 2004, pp. 131-154. Single or multiple copies of this article are available for a fee from The Haworth Document Delivery Service [1-800-HAWORTH, 9:00 a.m. - 5:00 p.m. (EST). E-mail address: docdelivery@haworthpress.com].

http://www.haworthpress.com/web/JHBSE
Digital Object Identifier: 10.1300/J137v10n01_02

Aspects of acculturation are measured both at the individual level (language used during interview and nativity) and couple level (dyad concordance on language preference and nativity). Multilevel analysis revealed significant correlation between spouses' depressive symptomatology (intraclass correlation, $\rho = .41$), suggesting that the study of depressive symptoms in MA couples requires attention to their interpersonal contexts. Contrary to expectation, acculturation, logged household size, and socioeconomic variables (education, logged household income, and logged household net worth wealth) were not significantly associated with depressive symptoms. Age and logged lower body disability were significantly associated with depressive symptoms. Discussion focuses on the importance and challenge of assessing acculturation when exploring risk and protective factors on depressive sympto- matology among mid-life and older MA couples. *[Article copies available for a fee from The Haworth Document Delivery Service: 1-800-HAWORTH. E-mail address: <docdelivery @haworthpress.com> Website: <http://www.HaworthPress.com> © 2004 by The Haworth Press, Inc. All rights reserved.]*

KEYWORDS. Acculturation, depression, couples, dyad research, Mexican American, Latino

INTRODUCTION

Acculturation, defined as a multidimensional, multidirectional, developmental, interactive, and adaptive process of cultural adjustments experienced by individuals (Cuellar, Arnold, & Maldonado, 1995; Padilla & Perez, 2003) and groups (Berry, 1997; Berry & Sam, 1996) across the life span, is considered pivotal in examining psychological distress in Hispanic persons.[1,2] The importance held by culture and social location, major components and correlates of acculturation, for understanding psychological distress is well-described (NIMH, 1995) and evidenced by the extent to which they are examined in relationship to depression, one of the most common emotional challenges found in older persons (Futterman, Thompson, Gallagher-Thompson, & Ferris, 1995), and the single most researched mental health outcome among Hispanic persons (Salgado de Snyder, 1987). Research that examines depressive symptomatology in older Mexican Americans (Aranda, Lee, & Wilson, 2001; Black, Markides, & Miller, 1998; González, Haan, & Hinton, 2001; Mills & Henretta, 2001), in particular, almost uniformly incorporates some aspect or measure of acculturation as a predictor or covariate. Irrespective of how aspects of acculturation are assessed, the major issue that is addressed in research that examines acculturation in relationship to depressive symptomatology is the extent that it increases or reduces risk for depression.

Results from studies that examine some aspect of acculturation and depressive symptomatology among samples including older Mexican Americans are somewhat equivocal. While some studies report an inverse relationship between some aspect of acculturation and depressive symptomatology (Black, Goodwin, & Markides, 1998; Garcia & Marks, 1988; González, Haan, & Hinton, 2001; Zamanian, Thackerey, Starrett, Brown, Lassman, & Blanchard, 1992), particularly where women are concerned (Black, Markides, & Miller, 1998; Black, Goodwin, & Markides, 1998; Kemp, Staples, Lopez-Aqueres, 1987), two studies report higher levels of depressive symptoms associated with higher acculturation (Golding & Burnam, 1990; Moscicki, Locke, Rae, & Boyd, 1989). Still other studies do not report detecting any relationship between certain aspects of acculturation, such as country of origin (Kemp, Staples, & Lopez-Aqueres, 1987) and depressive symptomatology. Inconsistent findings are also evident in research that examines aspects of acculturation and depressive symptomatology in younger, adult Mexican American persons (Alderete, Vega, Kolody, & Aguilar-Gaxiola, 1999; Cuellar & Roberts, 1997; Finch, Kolody, & Vega, 2000; Minuet-Vilaro, Folkman, & Gregorich, 1999).

One possible explanation for the discrepant findings in research that examines aspects of acculturation and depressive symptomatology in older persons is the distinct manner in which acculturation is measured across studies. The conceptual complexity of acculturation (for discussion on topic, see Berry, 1997; Cabassa, 2003; Chun, Organista, & Marin, 2003), which has yet to be captured in standardized instruments, encourages researchers to assess acculturation in terms of its more easily measured components or proxies. Language, in comparison to other acculturation indicators or proxies such as ethnicity, nativity (birth country) of self or parents, customs, and geographic residence, is considered the most potent factor in acculturation, and, as a result, is the factor most often assessed as an index or proxy of acculturation (Cuellar, Harris, & Jasso, 1980; Krause, Bennett, & Van Tran, 1989; Marin, Sabogal, VanOss, Otero-Sabogal, & Perez-Stable, 1987). Although formally not used as measures of social location, aspects of acculturation, such as language, nativity, and immigration status, are increasingly regarded as correlates of socioeconomic status (Finch,

Kolody, & Vega, 2000; Negy & Woods, 1992), rather than strictly components of acculturation.

Despite interest in examining the relationship between acculturation and depressive symptomatology in adult Mexican Americans, limited attention has been given to these concepts within the context of their marital environment. While the importance of examining acculturation and Mexican American couples is noted elsewhere (Negy & Snyder, 1997), only one study (Townsend, Miller, & Guo, 2001) is found that examines acculturation in relationship to depressive symptoms in Hispanic (Mexican Americans) married couples. Although a number of studies that examine acculturation and depressive symptomatology in adult Mexican Americans pay attention to marital status (Black, Markides, & Miller, 1998; Lopez-Aqueres, Kemp, Plopper, Staples, & Brummel-Smith, 1984; Mendes de Leon & Markides, 1988; Vega, Warheit, & Meinhardt, 1984), they strictly follow an individualistic orientation, that is, the individual is the preferred unit of conceptualization, measurement, and analysis.

In the only study found that examines depressive symptomatology within the context of Hispanic couples, namely Mexican American couples (Townsend, Miller, & Guo, 2001), findings confirm that both individual-level and couple-level covariates are important in explaining depressive symptomatology. Townsend, Miller, and Guo (2001) not only highlight the importance of the social context perspective, they cogently discuss the use of dyadic data and multilevel modeling to best understand depression in married couples. The authors suggest that acculturation and immigration history be examined in relationship to depressive symptomatology in Mexican Americans.

The paucity of basic and applied research that examines depressive symptoms within the social context of Mexican American couples is surprising. Mexican Americans are highly relational, as evidenced by their strong collective (Marin & Triandis, 1985) and family orientation (Angel & Angel, 1992; Markides, Boldt, & Ray, 1986; Markides & Martin, 1990; Sabogal, Marin, Otero-Sabogal, Marin, & Perez-Stable, 1987) and, therefore, are apt to share their psychological experiences with others within their immediate social contexts, such as spouses and partners. Ignoring social context when examining Mexican Americans not only dismisses their cultural inclination but yields biased results. The spectacular growth that Mexican Americans are experiencing, particularly older Mexican Americans who comprise the fastest growing subgroup both within and beyond the Hispanic community (U.S. Bureau of Census, 2000), in combination with their reported disproportionate levels of morbidity (National Institutes of Health, 2000), encourages the advancement of research approaches that generate the knowledge needed to best meet their health care needs.

The present study examines the role of acculturation in determining depressive symptomatology in adult, married Mexican American couples. This study assumes implicitly that the experience of depressive symptomatology among married persons is interdependent, as evidenced elsewhere (Barnett, Brennan, Marshall, Raudenbush, & Pleck, 1995; Bookwala & Schulz, 1996; Townsend, Miller, & Guo, 2001; Tower & Kasl, 1995; Whiffen & Aube, 1999). By focusing on Mexican American couples and capitalizing on multilevel statistical techniques that incorporate paired data as a focal part of the analysis, this study tests whether depressive symptoms covary within couples, whether the variability is significant (i.e., whether there are random effects) both within and between couples (Bryk & Raudenbush, 1992; Kreft & de Leeuw, 1998), and whether aspects of acculturation, adjusting for relevant covariates (i.e., age, years of formal education, logged lower body difficulties, logged household income, logged household net worth, logged household size), account for the variability. Two principal hypotheses are tested in this study: (1) depressive symptoms of wives and husbands will be significantly and substantially correlated; and, (2) low acculturation, while holding relevant variables constant (i.e., age, years of formal education, logged lower body difficulties, logged household income, logged household net worth, logged household size), will increase symptoms of depression.

The choice to examine the relevancy of the selected individual-level (lower body difficulty, age, education) and couple-level (household income, wealth, and size) control variables in this beginning examination of acculturation and depressive symptoms in the Latino marital environment is driven by prior research and data availability. Lower body difficulty was reasonable to include as a covariate in this study given the increasing documentation of a significant relationship between health-related indicators and depressive symptomatology in older Mexican Americans (Rodríguez Le Sage, 2002). Studies based on data from the Hispanic Established Population for the Epidemiologic Study of the Elderly (H-EPESE) alone, an ongoing National Institute on Aging-funded community-based study of 3,050 Mexican American subjects aged 65 and older (Markides, Rudkin, Angel, & Espino, 1997), report that high levels of depressive symptoms are significantly more common in older Latino persons with a number of functional impairments (Black, Goodwin, & Markides, 1998; Black, Markides, & Miller, 1998; Chiriboga,

Black, Aranda, & Markides, 2002). Another important study based on H-EPESE data reports a significant inverse relationship between baseline depressive symptoms score and physical performance score two years later (Raji, Ostir, Markides, & Goodwin, 2002).

The literature suggests that increased risk of high levels of depressive symptoms in older Latinos is associated with reported lower education achievement (Chiriboga, Black, Aranda, & Markides, 2002); lower or decreased income (Aranda, Lee, & Wilson, 2001; Chiriboga, Black, Aranda, Markides, 2002; Lopez-Aqueres, Kemp, Plopper, Staples, & Brummel-Smith, 1984; Kemp, Staples, & Lopez-Aqueres, 1987; Moscicki, Locke, Rae, & Boyd, 1989); and, being female (Aranda, Lee, & Wilson, 2001; Chiriboga, Black, Aranda, & Markides, 2002; González, Haan, & Hinton, 2001; Lopez-Aqueres, Kemp, Plopper, Staples, & Brummel-Smith, 1984). In addition, advancing age is reported to be significantly associated with high depressive symptoms in older Latinos (Mills & Henretta, 2001), yet it is suggested that this relationship may be associated with a transition to poor health and functional disability rather than to advancing old age itself. Finally, household size, an aspect of family solidarity, the special bond between family members particularly parents and adult children (Bengston & Schrader, 1982; Mangen & McChesney, 1988; Mangen, Bengston, & Landry,1988), was included in this study given reports that dimensions of inter- generational family solidarity are significantly associated with the psychological well-being of older Mexican Americans (Markides & Krause, 1985; Markides, Saldaña Costley, & Rodriguez, 1981; Markides & Martin, 1990).

METHOD

Design Sample

This study employs data from the Health and Retirement Survey (HRS), a large nationally representative panel study that is publicly available from the University of Michigan. Although the HRS is designed to meet multiple objectives, its general thrust is to better understand how aging affects noninstitutionalized persons over time. HRS began in 1992 with a multistage area probability sample of households in the contiguous United States, targeting all noninstitutionalized adults aged 51-61 years (i.e., born during the years 1931-1941) and spouses if married, regardless of age. Supplemental over-samples were drawn for

African Americans, Hispanics, and residents of the state of Florida. Initial interviews were conducted in person with mail/telephone interviews planned for every second year over 12 years. Interviews were conducted either in Spanish or English, depending on the participants' preference. The detailed description of the complex sample design is available through the HRS web site (University of Michigan, 2000).

The present analysis is based on Wave I (1992) of the HRS which consisted of 12,654 individuals and 7,600 households. The current sample was restricted to: (1) married couples in which both spouses identified themselves as having Mexican American origin; and, (2) couples who had complete data on all variables included in the analyses. Limiting the sample to married, Mexican American couples resulted preliminarily in 366 individuals (183 couples). Excluding an additional 20 individuals (10 couples) due to item nonresponse resulted in a final sample of 346 individuals comprising 173 couples.

This study's focus on Mexican American couples stems from practical and theoretical considerations. Mexican Americans not only comprise the largest subgroup in the Hispanic community (62%) (Therrien & Ramirez, 2000), but older Mexican Americans also comprise the fastest-growing older group both within and beyond the Hispanic community (U.S. Bureau of Census, 1996, 2000). In addition, understanding that Hispanic subgroups have unique ethnocultural orientations that may relate distinctly to how they experience environmental stressors and symptoms of depression (Krause & Goldenhar, 1992; NIMH, 1995), requires that Hispanic subgroups receive distinct attention. Finally, the small numbers of married couples in HRS representing varied Hispanic subgroups prevent across-group comparisons.

Measures

Table 1 summarizes the measures used in the present study. Additional details on measures follow.

Outcome: Depressive Symptomatology

Depressive symptomatology is assessed with a shortened version of the Center for Epidemiologic Studies Depression Scale (CES-D; Radloff, 1977). The shortened version of the CES-D individual-level index used in this study measures the occurrence and severity of eight symptoms related to depression (felt depressed, felt that everything was an effort, experienced restless sleep, was [not] happy, felt lonely, [did

TABLE 1. Measures

Individual-Level Outcome • Depressive symptomatology (8 CES-D items, scored low 8-32 high symptoms)
Individual-Level Predictors • Language (language used during interview: 0 = Spanish or 1 = English) • Nativity (birth country: 0 = Mexico or 1 = US) • Gender (0 = female or 1 = male) • Age (birth year subtracted from year of the interview) • Years of formal education (0 to 17+) • Number of lower body difficulties (LBD) (natural log of sum of 4 items involving: walking, climbing, pulling, lifting; score 0-4)
Couple-Level Predictors • Language concordance (0 = different language or 1 = same language) • Nativity concordance (0 = different nativity or 1 = same nativity) • Household Income (natural log of reported or imputed income measured in dollars) • Household Net Worth (natural log of reported or imputed net worth measured in   dollars) • Household Size (natural log of number of persons in the household)

not] enjoy life, could not get going) during the past week. Responses for negative symptoms are measured using a 4-point Likert rating (*1 = none or almost none of time, 2 = some of time, 3 = most of the time, 4 = all or almost all of the time*), with the values reversed for the positive items. The potential summed score ranges from 8 to 32, with the highest limit indicating greatest symptomatology. The eight items reflect three of four dimensions (depressed mood, lack of well-being, and psychomotor retardation) that underlie the original CES-D scale (Hertzog, 1989). In this study's sample, the eight items have good internal consistency (= .79). Both the original 20-item CES-D and modified versions of it have been used frequently with Latino adults across a broad age range, including mid-life and older Mexican Americans (Black, Markides, & Miller, 1998; Garcia & Marks, 1988; González, Haan, & Hinton, 2001; Mendes de Leon & Markides, 1988).

Individual-Level Predictors

Acculturation is measured both at the individual and couple levels. At the individual level, acculturation is assessed by language of the interview and nativity. Language of the interview is coded as a dichotomous variable: 0 = Spanish versus 1 = English. Thus, persons choosing to be interviewed in Spanish are the reference category and regarded as having low acculturation. Similarly, nativity is coded as a dichotomous variable: 0 = Mexico (born) versus 1 = US (born). Persons born in Mexico are the reference category and regarded as having low acculturation. Respondents were asked two questions to assess their nativity: "Were you born in the United States?"; and, if no, "In what country were you born?"

Age is calculated in years by subtracting the year of the participant's birth from the year of the interview, 1992. Education is measured in years, from 0 to 17 ($\geq$ 17), according to the highest grade of school or year of college that was completed. Gender is coded 0 = female or 1 = male.

Number of lower body difficulties (LBD) is assessed by adding reported number of lower body difficulties (walk several blocks, climb one flight of stairs without resting, pull or push large objects like a living room chair, lift or carry weights over 10 pounds like a heavy bag of groceries). In the present analyses, LBD is coded: 0 = not difficult versus 1 = difficult. Total scores, calculated by summing responses to all 4 items, can range from 0 to 4, with the highest limit indicating greatest number of lower body difficulties.

For multilevel analyses, age, education, and number of lower body difficulties are centered around their respective median values to facilitate the interpretation of results; the median age is 55, the median education level is sixth grade, and median LBD is 1.11. Thus, after centering, higher age levels represent age beyond 55 years, high scores on education represent education beyond sixth grade, and higher number of LBD represent number of LBD beyond 1.11. LBD was logged prior to centering.

Couple-Level Predictors

Aspects of acculturation at the couple level are assessed by couples' concordance on both their nativity and language of interview. Couple nativity concordance is coded as a dichotomous variable: 0 = Spouses with different nativity versus 1 = Spouses with same nativity. Thus, couples with each spouse having different nativity comprise the reference category. Couple language concordance is coded as a dichotomous variable: 0 = Spouses were interviewed in different languages versus 1 = Spouses were interviewed in same language. Hence, couples interviewed in different languages comprise the reference category.

Household size is measured as the number of persons in the household. Household income is measured as the total household income for the preceding year from all sources, including spouses' labor earnings, private pension and annuity income, disability and Social Security income, and income from other household members. Household net worth is measured as the total household, tangible, net worth in terms of both housing equity and non-housing equity (e.g., savings). Information on household income and household net worth either is reported by the spouse providing the household financial information or is imputed for the household. In terms of assessing household income, when the respondent is unable to provide exact amounts of income, they are asked to pick from a set of income categories.

For the multilevel analyses, logged values are calculated for household size, household income, and household net worth. In turn, these values are centered around their respective means to facilitate interpretation.

Analytical Approach

The analytical strategy included univariate and bivariate descriptive exploration followed by hierarchical linear modeling (HLM), optimally developed for analyses of hierarchical data, such as paired data from husbands and wives (Bryk & Raudenbush, 1992; Kreft & de Leeuw, 1998). Descriptive exploration was guided principally by paired t-test analysis for continuous variables and chi-square analysis for categorical variables. In turn, HLM was guided by two-level modeling based on an iterative generalized least squares estimation algorithm. To determine whether the second model represented a significant improvement in fit over the first model, the change in the value of -2 log likelihood function ($\Delta -2\ln L$; Kreft & de Leeuw, 1998) and the proportion reduction in "explainable" variance within couples (PRV_w) and between couples (PRV_b) (Bryk & Raudenbush, 1992) were used.

While descriptive data analysis was performed using the Statistical Package for Social Sciences (SPSS), multilevel analyses were performed using the Hierarchical Linear Modeling 5 program (Raudenbush, Bryk, Cheong, & Congdon, 2000). The significance level was set at $p \leq .05$. Relevant statistical assumptions of techniques employed were submitted to testing. The multilevel analyses incorporated weighted data that were adjusted for design effects.

The conceptual framework and flexible set of analytic tools available through HLM (Bryk & Raudenbush, 1992) permitted the examination of individual-level data clustered within aspects of the married couple context. There are several advantages in using HLM over simple random sampling (SRS) methods most commonly relied on by researchers who examine depression in married couples. Contrary to SRS methods that don't adjust to the interdependence of spousal data and, in turn, analyze the total sample covariance matrix and treat effects as fixed, HLM methods acknowledge the fact that spousal information is not independent, distinguish between the within-couple and between-couple covariance matrices, and allow for both fixed and random effects (Muthén, 1997). SRS methods, while subsuming variations across couples within random error, reduce the explanatory power of its models and don't take into account the importance of this variability (Raudenbush, 1995). In turn, HLM's clustering design permits corrected standard errors of estimate and, as a result, advances more accurate statistical inferences (Kreft & de Leeuw, 1998).

HLM 5 permitted testing this study's hypotheses with two nested models in which the intercept was specified as a random effect. Table 2 illustrates the multilevel equations that were modeled in this study.

To determine whether depressive symptomatology is correlated within couples and whether depressive symptom levels will vary both within couples and between couples, an initial model, with gender as the sole predictor (i.e., gender as a fixed effect), was tested. This model provides an estimate of the intraclass correlation (P) of depressive symptoms between spouses (representing the average association of depressive symptoms between spouses) and establishes whether between cou-

TABLE 2. Multi-Level Equations

Level 1: Y_{ij} (outcome [depressive symptoms] of individual i in couple j) =

$\beta_{oj} + \beta_{1j}(\text{Male}_{ij}) + \beta_{2j}(\text{Spanish}_{ij}) + \beta_{3j}(\text{Mexico}_{ij}) + \beta_{4j}(\text{LowerBodyDifficulty}_{ij})$

$+ \beta_{5j}(\text{Age}_{ij}) + \beta_{6j}(\text{Education}_{ij}) + r_{ij}$

Level 2: $\beta_{oj} = \gamma_{00} + \gamma_{01}(\text{Same Language}_j) + \gamma_{02}(\text{Same Nativity}_j) +$

$\gamma_{03}(\text{Household Income}_j) + \gamma_{04}(\text{Household Worth}_j) + \gamma_{05}(\text{Household Size}_j) + u_{oj}$

$\beta_{1j} = \gamma_{10}$ (average depressive symptoms of husbands)

$\beta_{2j} = \gamma_{20}$ (average depressive symptoms for everyone who is interviewed in English)

$\beta_{3j} = \gamma_{30}$ (average depressive symptoms for everyone born in the U.S.)

$\beta_{4j} = \gamma_{40}$ (average depressive symptoms for everyone with median logged lower body difficulty)

$\beta_{5j} = \gamma_{50}$ (average depressive symptoms for everyone with median age)

$\beta_{6j} = \gamma_{60}$ (average depressive symptoms for everyone with median education)

ple variability in depressive symptomatology is sufficiently present to justify further multilevel analysis (Bryk & Raudenbush, 1992).

To determine whether acculturation accounts for significant variability in depressive symptomatology, while adjusting for both individual-level and couple-level covariates, a second model was tested. This model included fixed individual effects of gender, two dichotomous variables representing acculturation (language of interview and nativity), age, education, and logged number of lower body difficulties; and fixed couple-level effects for two dichotomous variables representing acculturation at the couple level (nativity concordance and language concordance), logged household income, logged household net worth, and logged household size. Covariates were centered to facilitate interpretation of results (Bryk & Raudenbush, 1992). In each model, the intercept was specified as a random effect.

RESULTS

Bivariate Results

Table 3 presents descriptive data on all study measures for wives, husbands and couples, as well as paired t-test results (chi square analyses did not reveal any significant differences for categorical data). At the individual level, age, number of lower body difficulties, and number of depressive symptoms are significantly related to gender. Wives, on average, are significantly younger than husbands and report significantly more depressive symptoms and lower body difficulties than husbands. In terms of education, both wives and husbands report low mean levels of formal education completed that do not differ significantly from each other.

Aspects of acculturation, assessed both at the individual-level (language of interview and nativity) and couple-level (language and nativity concordance), are not meaningfully related to gender. The average household size of this sample is 4.14 persons, the average household income, $28,238, and the average household net worth, $94,863.

Hierarchical Linear Modeling Analyses

Correlation of symptom levels within couples and variability of symptoms between couples (Model 1). Table 4 presents the results of the hierarchical linear modeling. The variances of random effects in Model

TABLE 3. Individual/Couple-Level Descriptive Characteristics of Wives, Husbands, and Couples[a]

	Wives n = 173	Husbands n = 173	Couples n = 173
Depressive Symptoms** Mean±SD	13.12±4.35	11.48±3.87	
Age** Mean±SD	53.46±5.29	57.83±5.98	
Education Mean±SD	6.39±3.85	6.50±4.34	
Lower Body Difficulties** Mean±SD	1.28±1.37	.942±1.43	
Language n(%) English Spanish	76 (43.9) 97 (56.1)	75(43.4) 98(56.6)	
Nativity n(%) US Mexico	90(52.0) 83(48.0)	93(53.8) 80(46.2)	
Nativity Concordance n(%) Same Different			132(76.3) 41(23.7)
Language Concordance n(%) Same Lang Diff. Lang			142(82.1) 31(17.9)
Household Income Mean±SD			$28,238±$19,314
Household Net Worth Mean±SD			$94,863±$174,698
Household Size Mean±SD			4.14±1.85

[a]Sample includes married couples of Mexican American origin interviewed in the 1992 Health Retirement Survey (HRS), Wave I.
Significant gender difference: **p < .01

1 indicate significant variability in mean depression levels between couples (τ_{00}) and individuals (within couples, $\sigma2$). Consistent with this study's first hypothesis, strong intraclass correlation of depressive symptoms between spouses, calculated from results of HLM shown in Table 4, is revealed, $\rho = \tau_{00}/(\tau_{00} + \sigma2) = .41$, thus suggesting that 41% of the variance in depressive symptoms in one spouse can be explained by depressive symptoms of the second spouse.

The intercept in this model (γ_{00}) represents wives' mean depression level. As expected, wives' mean depression level(γ_{00}) is significantly

TABLE 4. Results for Initial and Final Multilevel Models in the HRS Married Mexican American Sample

Parameter Estimates	Model 1 (Gender Only)		Model 2 (All Predictors)	
	Coefficient	SE	Coefficient	SE
Intercept, γ_{00}	13.03***	0.31	11.14***	0.74
Individual-Level Covariates				
Male, γ_{10}	−1.57***	0.44	−0.80*	0.37
Spanish, γ_{20}			0.07	0.59
Mexico, γ_{30}			0.76	0.53
LowBodyDiff, γ_{40}			2.25***	0.32
Age, γ_{50}			−0.08*	0.04
Education, γ_{60}			−0.02	0.06
Couple-Level Covariates				
Same Language, γ_{01}			−0.46	0.68
Same Nativity, γ_{02}			0.29	0.60
Household Income, γ_{03}			−0.55	0.37
Household Worth, γ_{04}			0.06	0.70
Household Size, γ_{05}			0.22	0.15
Variances of Random Effects				
Couple-Level t_{00}	6.86***		5.15***	
Individual-Level, σ^2	9.76*		8.67*	
−2lnL	1920.60		1863.25	

Note. SE = standard error. −2lnL = value of the −2 log likelihood function. Education and age are centered around their respective medians (i.e., 6th grade and 55 years). Number of lower body difficulties (LowBodyDiff) is logged and centered around its median. Household income, household net worth, and household size are logged and centered around their respective means.
*p ≤ .05. ***p ≤ .001.

higher than that of husbands' mean depression level (γ_{10}). On average, the depression score for wives was 13.03 and the husbands', 11.46 (13.03 − 1.57 = 11.46).

Effects of acculturation while adjusting for both individual-level and couple-level covariates (Model 2). Model 2, which includes aspects of acculturation both at the individual and couple levels, as well as other individual-level and couple-level covariates, provides a significant improvement in fit over the initial model (Δ−2lnL = 57.35, Δ df =

10, $p < .01$). Including covariates results in an 11% reduction in variance within couples ($PRV_w = .112$) and a 25% reduction in variance between couples ($PRV_b = .248$). As previously noted, the proportion reduction in "explainable" variance within couples (PRV_w) and between couples (PRV_b) (Bryk & Raudenbush, 1992) is used to determine whether Model 2 represents a significant improvement in fit over Model 1.

The intercept in Model 2 represents the mean depression level of wives with median age, education, and logged lower body difficulties, mean logged household income, household net worth, and household size, who were born in the U.S., and who were interviewed in the English language. While three of six covariates at the individual level are significantly related to depressive symptomatology, none of the five covariates at the couple level are significantly related to depressive symptomatology. At the individual level, younger age (below the median), higher number of lower body difficulties (above the median), and being female are significant predictors of higher depressive symptomatology. Contrary to expectation, aspects of acculturation, as measured at individual and couple levels, and socioeconomic variables measured at individual (education) and couple levels (income, wealth, and household size), do not significantly predict depressive symptomatology.

DISCUSSION

The present study builds on the only study (Townsend, Miller, & Guo, 2001) found in the literature that includes a subsample of adult Mexican American couples in its examination of depressive symptomatology in married couples. Focusing on married, middle-aged and older, Mexican American couples who participated in the Health and Retirement Survey (HRS), Wave I, the present study examined how acculturation and other relevant factors influence depressive symptoms within the marital environment. Hierarchical linear modeling (Bryk & Raudenbush, 1992) permitted this study to apply a contextual framework and examine whether depressive symptoms covary within couples, whether the variability is significant and substantial, and whether aspects of acculturation, adjusting for relevant covariates, account for the variability.

The findings of this study support one hypothesis, namely, that depressive symptoms are significantly and substantially correlated between middle-aged and older, Mexican American spouses. Slightly more than two-fifths of the variance in depressive symptoms in one spouse was explained by the depressive symptoms of the second spouse. The substantial interdependence that was revealed suggests that results from studies that examine depression in Mexican Americans without taking their contexts into account are likely to lack important information and, therefore, be biased. In addition, the high correlation between Mexican American spouses suggests that optimal approaches to prevent and treat depression in Mexican Americans warrant added attention to the marital environment.

There are possible explanations for the significant clustering of depressive symptomatology between Mexican American husbands and wives. First, the cultural tendency for Mexican Americans to be collective in orientation and relational in practice (Marin & Triandis, 1985) is likely to encourage a reciprocal quality to depressive symptomatology in spouses. Second, middle-aged and older couples who share advancing age, along with a specific environment and life-style, may be jointly at risk for depressive symptoms. Third, persons with an inclination towards depressive symptoms may tend to select mates who have a similar inclination. Finally, it is possible that the demands of one spouse's depressive symptoms engender depressive symptoms in the second spouse as well.

Besides discovering that depressive symptomatology was substantially correlated between spouses, the results revealed that several individual-level variables, but no couple-level variables, helped explain some of the variability in depression level. The finding that women reported, on average, a higher level of depressive symptomatology in comparison to men is consistent with previous research that compares gender differences in depressive symptomatology in older Mexican American persons (Aranda, Lee, & Wilson, 2001; Black, Markides, & Miller, 1998; González, Haan, & Hinton, 2001; Townsend, Miller, & Guo, 2001). The finding that the number of lower body difficulties predicted depressive symptomatology supports other studies of older Mexican Americans that report the influence of chronic conditions and functional impairment on depressive symptomatology (Black, Goodwin, & Markides, 1998; Chiriboga, Black, Aranda, & Markides, 2002; Raji, Ostir, Markides, & Goodwin, 2002; Snih, Markides, Ray, & Goodwin, 2001).

Contrary to expectation, aspects of acculturation as measured both at the individual-level and couple-level were not significantly associated with depressive symptoms. Thus, participants' nativity, language in which they were interviewed, or whether they shared the same language of the interview and nativity with their spouses did not help explain depressive symptoms. Furthermore, household size and socioeconomic status (e.g., education, income, and wealth), known correlates of acculturation (Negy & Woods, 1992a), were not significantly associated to depressive symptoms in this study.

Why acculturation was not associated with depressive symptoms is unclear and can only be speculated. A possible explanation may be that the assessment of acculturation lacked the sensitivity necessary to demonstrate subtle cultural differences. This study's examination of only two aspects or proxies of acculturation, language of interview and nativity, perhaps ignored other aspects of the acculturation process that are more important in explaining depressive symptoms. A third aspect of acculturation that is assessed by HRS but not examined in the present study, year of immigration, may be worthwhile to examine in future HRS-based studies that examine acculturation in relationship to depressive symptomatology in Mexican American couples.

The major justification for assessing acculturation in like manner, other than one of pragmatics in yielding to available measures of secondary data, is that language is considered the most potent factor in acculturation (Cuellar, Harris, & Jasso, 1980; Krause, Bennett, & Van Tran, 1989). In addition, others have noted that language (Negy & Woods, 1992b; Vega, Zimmerman, Gil, Warheit, & Apospori, 1993) and generation status are the most commonly used indices of acculturation (Negy & Woods, 1992b).

Nonetheless, there are problems associated with strictly relying on language used in an interview, or even language preference and nativity to assess acculturation. Language used in the interview does not truly reflect language preference or language proficiency, as persons can be proficient in several languages and use them selectively. In addition, learning a second language does not indicate the extent to which values associated with that linguistic tradition are adopted. Finally, assuming that United States' nativity is logically related to increases in acculturation, ignores the transnational experience of many U.S.-Mexico border residents who, despite being born in the United States or having lived here for many generations, prefer to speak Spanish and have a strong Mexican culture orientation.

While the use of tested acculturation scales may ensure that aspects of acculturation, such as language preference, language pattern use, nativity, generation status, and ethnicity, are more fully assessed, the problem of under-conceptualizing and under-measuring acculturation remains. The more popular acculturation scales, such as the Short Acculturation Scale for Hispanics (Marin, Sabogal, VanOss, Otero-Sabogal, & Perez-Stable, 1987), the Acculturation Rating Scale for Mexican Americans (ARSMA; Cuellar, Harris, & Jasso, 1980), the Revised ARSMA (Cuellar, Arnold, & Maldonado, 1995), and the Acculturation Scale developed by Hazuda, Haffner, and Stern (1988), focus heavily on language preference and patterns. Other scales that assess values and attitudes, such as the Measure of Acculturation developed by Flores-Ortiz, Coyne, and Mesa (Flores-Ortiz, 1991), remain under-tested and, hence, underused.

The importance of acculturation in understanding social and psychological distress in Mexican Americans demands advancing its conceptualization and measurement. While the complex nature of acculturation and the contextual factors that influence it (Berry, 1997; Berry & Sam, 1996; Hardwood, 1994) may preclude ever having a scale capable of adequately and sufficiently capturing it, the development of multiple measures that assess distinct aspects of acculturation will improve the validity and generalizability of study findings. As noted elsewhere (Espino & Maldonado, 1990), besides developing newer, standardized instruments to assess acculturation in Mexican Americans, uniform use of acculturation measures would make acculturation studies on older Mexican Americans more comparable and reproducible. In the absence of acculturation measures that adequately capture the multi-level changes that are experienced in the acculturation process of different Hispanic groups, research is likely to continue to simplify acculturation to a single domain (e.g., language use and preference, ethnic loyalty, cultural awareness, generation status, and nativity) for pragmatic reasons.

Other important limitations of this study, besides those associated with the measurement of acculturation, should be noted. A major shortcoming of this study is that it is cross-sectional and as such does not examine the potential effect that both individual and couple-level predictors may have on depressive symptomatology over time. Because certain processes, such as acculturation, can take a long time to unfold and distinctly impact marriages over time (Krause & Goldenhar, 1992), the examination of the long-term effects of acculturation on depressive symptomatology in couples is warranted. Longitudinal examination of intra-class correlation will help clarify whether the interdependence in depressive symptoms persists over time.

Another important limitation in this study is that the sample is small and restricted to married couples whose spouses are Mexican American. Findings are not generalizable to other couples such as cohabiting Mexican American couples who are not married, including gay and lesbian couples, and inter-ethnic couples in which only one spouse or partner is Mexican American. Excluding couples who have distinct orientations to marriage and partnering ignores factors that can potentially influence the nature of couples' interdependence.

Despite this study's shortcomings, the results provide encouraging evidence that may have a role in future research and clinical work related to depressive symptomatology in middle-aged and older, married, Mexican American couples. The present study stresses the importance of the interdependent nature of depressive symptoma- tology in Mexican American couples and illustrates the advantages of relational-based inquiry. It supports the growing body of evidence that depression levels within marital environment are relational (Barnett, Brennan, Marshall, Raudenbush, & Pleck, 1995; Bookwala & Schulz, 1996; Townsend, Miller, & Guo, 2001; Tower & Kasl, 1995; Whiffen & Aube, 1999). The study contributes to the very small existing literature on Mexican American couples rather than individuals.

NOTES

1. The terms *Hispanic* and *Mexican American* (MA) are not preferred by all members of the ethnic group and subgroup they intend to represent. In order to eliminate potential confusion by using other terms interchangeably (e.g., *Latino* for *Hispanic* or *Chicano* and *Mexicano* for *Mexican American*), the terms *Hispanic* and *Mexican American* will be used throughout the article to refer to persons who have Spanish origins and Mexican/Chicano origins, respectively.

2. While acculturation involves both individual-level and group-level phenomena as a result of culturally-distinct groups interacting continuously with one another on a first-hand basis, individual-level adaptation has received the most attention. Literature addressing acculturation most often refers to a process of change that members of a minority group experience toward the adoption of a majority culture; rarely is acculturation discussed in reference to majority group members adapting into an ethnic or minority subculture. Nonetheless, conceptual analysis of acculturation has been developing steadily to advance our understanding of the direction that the process may take (e.g., movement from adherence to the culture of origin and immersion to the dominant culture or maintenance of culture of origin and adherence to the dominant or host culture), contextual factors that influence the acculturation process (e.g., home and host environments), and adaptation responses to the process (e.g., stress/distress coping strategies).

REFERENCES

Alderete, E., Vega, W. A., Kolody, B., & Aguilar-Gaxiola, S. (1999). Depressive symptomatology: Prevalence and psychosocial risk factors among Mexican migrant farmworkers in California. *Journal of Community Psychology, 27*(4), 457-471.

Angel, J. L., & Angel, R. J. (1992). Age at migration, social connections, and well-being among elder Hispanics. *Journal of Aging Health, 4*, 480-499.

Aranda, M. P., Lee, P. J., & Wilson, S. (2001). Correlates of depression in older Latinos. *Home Health Care Services Quarterly, 20*(1), 1-20.

Barnett, R. C., Raudenbush, S. W., Brennan, R. T., Pleck, J. H., & Marshall, N. L. (1995). Change in job and marital experiences and change in psychological distress: A longitudinal study of dual-earner couples. *Journal of Personality and Social Psychology, 69*(5), 839-850.

Bengston, V. L., & Schrader, S. (1982). Parent-child relations. In D. J. Mangen & W. A. Peterson (Eds.), *Research instruments in social gerontology* (Vol. 2, pp. 115-186). Minneapolis: University of Minnesota Press.

Berry, J. W. (1997). Immigration, acculturation, and adaptation. *Applied Psychology: An International Review, 46*(1), 5-33.

Berry, J. W., & Sam, D. L. (1996). Acculturation and adaptation. In J. W. Berry, M. A. Segall, & C. Kagitubasi (Eds.), *Handbook of cross-cultural psychology: Social behaviors and application* (Vol. 3, pp. 291-326). Boston: Allyn & Bacon.

Black, S. A., Goodwin, J. S., & Markides, K. S. (1998). The association between chronic diseases and depressive symptomatology in older Mexican Americans. *Journal of Gerontology, 53A*(3), M188-M194.

Black, S. A., Markides, K. S., & Miller, T. Q. (1998). Correlates of depressive symptomatology among older community-dwelling Mexican Americans: The Hispanic EPESE. *Journal of Gerontology, 53B*, S198-S208.

Bookwala, J., & Schulz, R. (1996). Spousal similarity in subjective well-being: The cardiovascular health study. *Psychology and Aging, 11*(4), 582-590.

Bryk, A., & Raudenbush, S. (1992). *Hierarchical linear models: Applications and data analysis methods.* Newbury Park, CA: Sage.

Cabassa, L. J. (2003). Measuring acculturation: Where we are and where we need to go. *Hispanic Journal of Behavioral Sciences, 25*, 127-146.

Chiriboga, D. A., Black, S. A., Aranda, M., & Markides, K. (2002). Stress and depressive symptoms among Mexican American elders. *Journal of Gerontology: Psychological Sciences, 57B*(6), P559-568.

Chun, K. M., Organista, P. B., & Marin, G. (Eds.) (2003). *Acculturation: Advances in theory, measurement, and applied research.* Washington, DC: American Psychological Association.

Codina, G. E., & Montalvo, F. F. (1994). Chicano phenotype and depression. *Hispanic Journal of Behavioral Sciences, 16*(3), 296-306.

Cuellar, I., & Roberts, R. E. (1997). Relations of depression, acculturation, and socioeconomic status in a Latino sample. *Hispanic Journal of Behavioral Sciences, 19*(2), 230-238.

Cuellar, I., Harris, L. C., & Jasso, R. (1980). An acculturation scale for Mexican American normal and clinical populations. *Hispanic Journal of Behavioral Sciences*, 2, 199- 217.

Cuellar, I., Arnold, B., & Maldonado, R. (1995). Acculturation Rating Scale for Mexican Americans–II: A revision of the original ARSMA Scale. *Hispanic Journal of Behavioral Sciences*, 17, 275-304.

Espino, D., & Maldonado, D. (1990). Hypertension and acculturation in elderly Mexican Americans: Results from 1982-84 Hispanic HANES. *Journal of Gerontology*, 45(6), M209-213.

Finch, B. K., Kolody, B., & Vega, W. (2000). Perceived discrimination and depression among Mexican-origin adults in California. *Journal of Health and Social Behavior*, 41, 295-313.

Flores-Ortiz, Y. G. (1991). Levels of acculturation, marital satisfaction, and depression among Chicana workers: A psychological perspective. *Aztlan*, 20(1 & 2), 151-175.

Futterman, A., Thompson, L., Gallagher-Thompson, D., & Ferris, R. (1995). Depression in later life: Epidemiology, assessment, etiology, and treatment. In E.E. Beckham & W.R. Leber (Eds.), *Handbook of depression* (2nd ed.) (pp. 494-525). New York: Guilford.

Garcia, M., & Marks, G. (1988). Depressive symptomatology among Mexican American adults: An examination with the CES-D scale. *Psychiatry Research*, 27, 137-148.

Golding, J., & Burnam, A. (1990). Immigration, stress, and depressive symptoms in a Mexican American community. *Journal of Nervous Mental Disorder*, 178(3), 161-171.

González, H. M., Haan, M. N., & Hinton, L. (2001). Acculturation and the prevalence of depression in older Mexican Americans: Baseline results of the Sacramento area of Latino study on aging. *Journal of the American Geriatrics Society*, 49, 948-953.

Hazuda, H. P., Haffner, S. M., & Stern, M. P. (1988). Acculturation and assimilation among Mexican Americans: Scales and population-based data. *Social Science Quarterly*, 69, 687-705.

Hertzog, C. (1989). Using confirmatory factor analysis for scale development and validation. In M. P. Lawton, & A. R. Hertzog (Eds.), *Special research methods for gerontology* (pp. 281-306), Amityville, NY: Baywood.

Kemp, B. J., Staples, F., & Lopez-Aqueres, W. (1987). Epidemiology of depression and dysphoria in an elderly Hispanic population. *Journal of American Geriatrics Society*, 35, 920-926.

Krause, N., Bennett, J., & Van Tran, T. (1989). Age difference in the acculturation process. *Psychology and Aging*, 4, 321-332.

Krause, N., & Goldenhar, L. M. (1992). Acculturation and psychological distress in three groups of elderly Hispanics. *Journal of Gerontology*, 47(6), S279-S288.

Kreft, I., & de Leeuw, J. (1998). *Introducing multilevel modeling*. Thousand Oaks, CA: Sage.

Lopez-Aqueres, W., Kemp, B., Plopper, M., Staples, F. R., & Brummel-Smith, K. (1984). Health needs of the Hispanic elderly. *Journal of Geriatrics Society*, 32, 191-198.

Mangen, D. J., Bengston, V. L., & Landry, P. H. (1988). *Measurement intergenerational relations*. Beverly Hills: Sage.

Mangen, D. J., & McChesney, K. Y. (1988). Intergenerational cohesion: A comparison of linear and nonlinear analytical approaches. *Research on Aging, 1*, 121-136.

Marin, G., Sabogal, F., VanOss, B., Otero-Sabogal, R., & Perez-Stable, E. (1987). Development of a short acculturation scale for Hispanics. *Hispanic Journal of Behavioral Sciences, 9*(2), 183-205.

Marin, G., & Triandis, H. C. (1985). Allocentrism as an important characteristic of the behavior of Latin Americans and Hispanics. In R. Diaz-Guerrero (Ed.), *Cross-cultural and national studies in social psychology* (pp. 85-104). Amsterdam: Elsevier Science.

Markides, K. S., Boldt, J. S., & Ray, L. A. (1986). Sources of helping and intergenerational solidarity: A three-generation study of Mexican Americans. *Journal of Gerontology, 41*(4), 506-511.

Markides, K. S., & Krause, N. (1985). Intergenerational solidarity and psychological well-being among older Mexican Americans: A three-generations study. *Journal of Gerontology, 40*, 390-392.

Markides, K. S., & Martin, H. W. (1990). *Older Mexican Americans: Selected findings from two San Antonio studies.* San Antonio, TX: Tomas Rivera Center.

Markides, K. S., Rudkin, L., Angel, R. J., & Espino, D. V. (1997). Health status of Hispanic elderly. In L. J. Martin & B. Soldo (Eds.), *Racial and ethnic differences in the health of older Americans* (pp. 285-300). Washington, DC: National Academy Press.

Markides, K. S., Saldaña Costley, D., & Rodriguez, L. (1981). Perceptions of intergenerational relations and psychological well-being among elderly Mexican Americans: A causal model. *International Journal of Aging and Human Development, 13*, 43-52.

Mendes de Leon, C. F., & Markides, K. (1988). Depressive symptoms among Mexican Americans: A three generation study. *American Journal of Epidemiology, 127*(1), 150-160.

Mills, T. L., & Henretta, J. C. (2001). Racial, ethnic, and sociodemographic differences in the level of psychosocial distress among older Americans. *Research on Aging, 23*(2), 131-152.

Minuet-Vilaro, F., Folkman, S., & Gregorich, S. (1999). Depressive symptomatology in three Latino groups. *Western Journal of Nursing Research, 21*(2), 209-224.

Moscicki, E. K., Locke, B. Z., Rae, D. S., & Boyd, J. H. (1989). Depressive symptoms among Mexican Americans: The Hispanic health and nutrition examination survey. *American Journal of Epidemiology, 130*(2), 348-360.

Muthén, B. (1997). Latent variable modeling of longitudinal and multilevel data. In A. Raftery (Ed.), *Sociological methodology* (pp. 453-480). Boston: Blackwell.

National Institute of Mental Health (NIMH) (1995). *Basic behavioral science research for mental health: A report of the National Advisory Mental Health Council* (NIH Publication N. 95-3682). Washington, DC: U.S. Government Printing Office.

National Institutes of Health (NIMH) (2000, October). *National Institutes of Health Strategic Plan to Reduce and Ultimately Eliminate Health Disparities, Fiscal Years 2002-2006.* Bethesda, MD: U.S. Department of Health and Human Services. *http://www.nih.gov/about/* (then click on Health Disparities).

Negy, C., & Snyder, D. K. (1997). Ethnicity and acculturation: Assessing Mexican American couples' relationships using the marital satisfaction inventory–revised. *Psychological Assessment, 9*(4), 414-421.

Negy, C., & Woods, D. J. (1992a). A note on the relationship between acculturation and socioeconomic status. *Hispanic Journal of Behavioral Sciences, 14*(2), 248-251.

Negy, C., & Woods, D. J. (1992b). The importance of acculturation in understanding research with Hispanic-Americans. *Hispanic Journal of Behavioral Sciences, 14*(2), 224-247.

Padilla, A. M., & Perez, W. (2003). Acculturation, social identity, and social cognition: A new perspective. *Hispanic Journal of Behavioral Sciences, 25*(1), 35-55.

Radloff, L. (1977). The CES-D Scale: A self-report depression scale for research in the general population. *Applied Psychological Measurement, 1*, 385-401.

Raji, M. A., Ostir, G. V., Markides, K. S., & Goodwin, J. S. (2002). The interaction of cognitive and emotional status on subsequent physical functioning in older Mexican Americans: Findings from the Hispanic Established Population for the Epidemiologic Study of the Elderly. *Journal of Gerontology: Medical Sciences, 57A*(10), M678-M682.

Raudenbush, S. (1995). Hierarchical linear models to study the effects of social context on development. In J. Gottman (Ed.), *The analysis of change* (pp. 165-201). Mahwah, NJ: Lawrence Erlbaum Associates.

Raudenbush, S., Bryk, A., Cheong, Y. F., & Congdon, R. (2000). *HLM5: Hierarchical Linear and Nonlinear Modeling.* Lincolnwood, IL: Scientific Software International, Inc.

Rodríguez Le Sage, M. (2002, November). Association Between Health Indicators and Depressive Symptomatology in Mexican American Couples. Paper presented at the 55th Annual Scientific Meeting of the Gerontological Society of America, Washington, DC.

Sabogal, F., Marin, G., Otero-Sabogal, R., Marin, B. V., & Perez-Stable, E. J. (1987). Hispanic familism and acculturation: What changes and what doesn't? *Hispanic Journal of Behavioral Sciences, 9*(4), 397-412.

Salgado de Snyder, V. N. (1987). Factors associated with acculturative stress and depressive symptomatology among married Mexican immigrant women. *Psychology of Women Quarterly, 11*, 475-488.

Snih, S. A., Markides, K. S., Ray, L., & Goodwin, J. S. (2001). Impact of pain on disability among older Mexican Americans. *Journal of Gerontology: Medical Sciences, 56A*(7), M400-M404.

Stroup-Benham, C. A., Markides, K. S., Black, S. A., & Goodwin, J. S. (2000). Relationship between low blood pressure and depressive symptomatology in older people. *Journal of American Geriatrics Society, 48*, 250-255.

Therrien, M., & Ramirez, R. R. (2000). The Hispanic population in the United States: March 2000. *Current population reports* (Publication No. P20-535). Washington, DC: U.S. Bureau of the Census.

Tower, R. B., & Kasl, S. (1995). Depressive symptoms across older spouses and the moderating effect of marital closeness. *Psychology and Aging, 10*(4), 625-638.

Townsend, A. L., Miller, B., & Guo, S. (2001). Depression in middle-aged and older married couples: A dyadic analysis. *Journal of Gerontology, Social Sciences, 56B*, 5352-5361.

University of Michigan. Health and Retirement Study Overview (updated July 1999). Retrieved May 23, 2000, from *http://www.umich.edu/~hrswww/overview/hrsover. html*.

U.S. Bureau of Census (1996). *Population projections of the U.S. by age, sex, race, and Hispanic origin: 1995 to 2050.* Washington, DC: U.S. Government Printing Office.

U.S. Bureau of Census (2000). *Estimates of the U.S. by race and Hispanic origin.* Washington, DC: U.S. Government Printing Office.

Vega, W., Zimmerman, R., Gil, A., Warheit, G., & Apospori, E. (1993). Acculturative strain theory: Its application in explaining drug use behavior among Cuban and non-Cuban Hispanic youth. In M. DeLaRosa (Ed.), *Drug Abuse Among Minority youth: Advances in research and methodology* (pp. 144-166). Rockville, MD: National Institute of Drug Administration.

Vega, W. A., Warheit, G .J., & Meinhardt, K. (1984). Marital disruption and the prevalence of depressive symptomatology among Anglos and Mexican Americans. *Journal of Marriage and Family*, 817-874.

Whiffen, V. E., & Aube, J. A. (1999). Personality, interpersonal context and depression in couples. *Journal of Social and Personal Relationships, 16*(3), 369-383.

Zamanian, K., Thackerey, M., Starrett, R. A., Brown, L. G., Lassman, D. K., & Blanchard, A. (1992). Acculturation and depression in Mexican American elderly. *Clinical Gerontologist, 11*(3-9), 109-121.

SPIRITUALITY

Meeting Life Challenges:
A Hierarchy of Coping Styles
in African American
and Jewish American Older Adults

Holly B. Nelson-Becker

SUMMARY. Mental health and social service providers need to understand the contextual experience of diverse aging populations and the types of life challenges they have encountered. This research examined

Holly Nelson-Becker, PhD, is Assistant Professor and Hartford Faculty Scholar in Geriatric Social Work, School of Social Welfare, The University of Kansas, 1545 Lilac Lane, Lawrence, KS 66044 (E-mail: hnelson@ku.edu).
The author thanks Dr. Rosemary Chapin, Dr. Berit Ingersoll-Dayton, and Dr. Theresa Koenig for comments on earlier versions of this paper. The author also thanks the Council for Jewish Elderly, Chicago, Illinois, for granting permission to include their clients in this study.

The research was supported by a dissertation grant from University of Chicago, School of Social Service Administration.

[Haworth co-indexing entry note]: "Meeting Life Challenges: A Hierarchy of Coping Styles in African American and Jewish American Older Adults." Nelson-Becker, Holly B. Co-published simultaneously in *Journal of Human Behavior in the Social Environment* (The Haworth Social Work Practice Press, an imprint of The Haworth Press, Inc.) Vol. 10, No. 1, 2004, pp. 155-174; and: *Diversity and Aging in the Social Environment* (eds: Sherry M. Cummings, and Colleen Galambos) The Haworth Social Work Practice Press, an imprint of The Haworth Press, Inc., 2004, pp. 155-174. Single or multiple copies of this article are available for a fee from The Haworth Document Delivery Service [1-800-HAWORTH, 9:00 a.m. - 5:00 p.m. (EST). E-mail address: docdelivery@haworthpress.com].

Digital Object Identifier: 10.1300/J137v10n01_03   *155* the life challenges specified by a purposive sample of 75 urban community-dwelling low-income older adults from four high-rise housing facilities. Thirty-four study participants were Jewish American and 41 were African American. Results indicate that many participants of both groups identified personal events such as bereavement and health as stressors, but only the Jewish Americans identified societal events such as World War II. Both groups found social resources moderately valuable in meeting life challenges, but religious resources were frequently identified by African American older adults and personal resources were highly endorsed by Jewish Americans, resulting in a hierarchy of coping styles for each group. Results suggest that mental health and social service providers can create interventions to reinforce and strengthen natural client resources that may vary according to ethnic and racial differences *[Article copies available for a fee from The Haworth Document Delivery Service: 1-800-HAWORTH. E-mail address: <docdelivery@ haworthpress.com> Website: <http://www.HaworthPress.com> © 2004 by The Haworth Press, Inc. All rights reserved.]*

KEYWORDS. Older adults, stress and coping, problem-solving, life challenge, ethnicity, African Americans, Jewish Americans, religion

INTRODUCTION

In an increasingly multicultural society, social workers and other mental health practitioners interact with clients who have different cultural backgrounds from their own. A multicultural stance to practice encourages the clinician to seek out and apply information on racial and ethnic minorities while at the same time developing a habit of inquiry. It is important to understand how cultural differences may affect the ways minority older adults respond to life challenges. Coping with life challenge and change is of particular concern to gerontological social workers who specialize in all aspects of the helping process (Bjorck & Cohen, 1993; Hooyman & Kiyak, 2002; McInnis-Dittrich, 2002; Miley, O'Melia, & DuBois, 2001). Developing a deeper understanding of how minority older adults both appraise and manage life challenge will assist helping professionals to move beyond assumptions about treatment to design interventions targeted to resources that will not only be accepted, but embraced.

A heuristic approach to knowledge asks how variables of race and ethnicity relate to coping processes. Qualitative research methods that employ a heuristic approach allow researchers to overcome the limitations of assumptions inherent in fixed choice questionnaires, while quantitative research methods provide information about prevalence that qualitative designs alone cannot. This paper reviews the stress and coping literature and describes a background conceptual model. Qualitative and quantitative data are presented on the life challenges and responses identified by two groups of ethnically and racially diverse older adults, African Americans and Jewish Americans. A hierarchy of coping styles that emerged from the data is presented and implications for research and practice are discussed.

LIFE CHALLENGES

Stress and Coping

The stress and coping paradigm has been a frequently used framework for understanding late-life adaptation (Kahana et al, 1999). Older adults face normative challenges in the form of bereavement, health problems, and relationship difficulties that highlight lack of congruence between person and environment. A critical life events approach to measuring stress identifies the event as a discrete change in a person's environment that is externally confirmable and requires a response (Billings & Moos, 1981; Jones & Kinman, 2001). A life event may be defined as unexpected, falling outside the parameters of everyday experience unlike daily hassles and uplifts (Lazarus & Folkman, 1989). Life events can subsume crises such as diagnosis of cancer or unanticipated death of a spouse. By contrast, chronic conditions may include stressors that are always present but not appraised as consistently difficult. A caregiving relationship in which an older adult provides care to an even older relative and experiences the vacillating benefits/costs is one example of a chronic stressor. Stress is the perceived outcome of an imbalance where the care receiver may require more than the care provider can easily give.

These critical life events and chronic conditions, defined in this paper as life challenges, motivate an active or passive behavioral reaction (Gottlieb, 1997; Snyder, 2001; Zeidner & Endler, 1996). Kahana et al. (1995) emphasize that life events and chronic conditions provide contexts of mutual interpretation among actors that may or may not result in appraisal of stress overload. In other words, such factors as the presence of social support may moderate the stressor. Stress requires a response to either alter the nature of the situation or one's response to it (Lazarus & Folkman, 1984). The former is referred to as problem-focused coping and the latter as emotion-focused coping. Problem-focused coping or instrumental coping is thus oriented toward an action stance. The goal is to ameliorate the underlying problem by solving it or minimizing its effects. By contrast, emotion-focused coping consists of cognitive restructuring to reduce emotional distress, not to change or eliminate the problem.

Race and Life Challenges

There has been much discussion in the literature regarding the benefits and disadvantages of ethnic, racial, and cultural factors in regard to stress and coping with the challenges of aging (Jackson, Chatters, & Taylor, 1993; Zeidner & Endler, 1996). Race in particular may be seen as either a biological or a social variable. As a social variable, race may shape interpersonal interaction due to power differential and class categorizations, or stereotypes, made by either party (Fiske, 1993). Race and ethnicity may be used to self-limit choices or to constrain the array of socially acceptable choices made in response to problems. The complex social components of race and ethnicity require further research to understand how they affect older adults and their needs. Some researchers argue that minority elders are doubly disadvantaged when they face late life due to the stressors of aging and minority status, particularly if they encounter discrimination (Binstock & George, 1990). Others suggest that minority older adults have developed unique strengths based on the lifetime challenges they have experienced that serve to bolster individual adaptation (Hooyman & Kiyak, 1999).

Religious involvement and family support are important sources of adaptive coping for African Americans. Ellison and Taylor (1996) reported that in an African American sample prayer was used often with health problems and bereavement. Although the family is a primary source of support for African American older adults as it is for other older adults, African Americans tend to receive help from multiple family members and have a more varied network that extends beyond the immediate family to distant relatives and friends (Bowles et al., 2000).

American Jewish culture has not been investigated to an equal extent, though historically Jewish Americans, too, have been marginalized in society. As Myerhoff (1992) noted, this ethnic group often expressed values of endurance and cultural inventiveness as they faced life challenge. While conducting an ethnographic study of aging at a senior center in Venice, California, Myerhoff described center members' struggles with extreme poverty, poor health, and loss of social roles. Through ingenuity, imagination, and boldness, this Jewish group of older adults rejected their social invisibility by taking on new roles in the center community.

Although general research on stress and coping in African American elders has been conducted (Cantor, Brennan, & Sainz, 1994; Ellison & Taylor, 1996; Jackson, Chatters, & Taylor, 1993), little is known about what supports they turn to first, what hierarchy of coping styles might inform mental health practice. There is a gap in knowledge about ways Jewish American elders cope with change. The current study addresses this gap by exploring the strategies these two ethnic and racial minority groups apply in meeting life challenges. These groups were chosen as the focus for this study because they have both been marginalized in American society. This research broadens social work knowledge about the process of coping and the types of natural supports that African American and Jewish American older adults may seek to age in place, assisting professionals to help strengthen present coping styles and possibly generate new ones.

METHOD

Sampling for this mixed-method qualitative and quantitative study was purposive and incorporated four low-income high-rise older adult housing sites in a large mid-western metropolitan area. The interviewer approached every individual who entered the apartment lobby at each site over a two-hour span during varying times of day to explain the study and arrange appointments for those interested. A small monetary incentive was offered at the completion of interviews. The study was approved by two IRBs, one affiliated with a university and one with a community organization that facilitated client access to two of the four sites. Interviews commenced with open-ended questions to distinguish the types of life challenge participants faced and to determine what type of coping responses they employed. A similar design had been used previously by Koenig (1995) who asked a sample of veterans how they coped with stress. Later interview questions asked participants to define religion and spirituality and whether they typically made a distinction between these terms, to state how important each domain was, and to identify in what specific ways they had used religion and spirituality to solve problems.

Participants in the study were asked demographic questions that included religious affiliation and frequency of church attendance. Three standardized scales were also administered: the Geriatric Depression Scale (Yesavage, Brink, Rose, & Leirer, 1983), the Life Satisfaction Index (Neugarten, Havighurst, & Tobin, 1961), and the Problem Solving Inventory (Heppner & Petersen, 1982). In addition, the author field-tested a new instrument, the Spiritual Strategies Scale (Nelson-Becker, 1999). Questions were administered orally and interviews ranged in length from one to two-and-one-half hours. Interviews were audiotaped and transcribed.

In the analysis, data was reconstructed into categories as emerging patterns developed using constant comparative analysis in the grounded theory approach of Glaser and Strauss (1967). Trustworthiness is a key consideration for achieving rigor in qualitative analysis: verification occurred through checking for distortions in communication with study participants and completing a coding check with a second rater. This paper reports on the data concerning life challenges and concomitant coping responses provided by the first questions mentioned above.

RESULTS

Sample

This study was based on a sample of 75 low-income community-dwelling older adults. It had a 91% participation rate. Thirty-four individuals participated from two Jewish American sites and 41 from two African American sites. The four sites were nearly racially segregated with two exceptions. One respondent in the African American sites was Jewish and one respondent in the primarily Jewish sites was African American.

The majority of respondents were women (n = 63) with 12 men, nearly evenly distributed across ethnic groups. Ages ranged from 58-92, with a median age of 81 in the Jewish American group and 75 in the African American group. Median educational level was the same for both groups at 12 years. Ninety-six percent of the entire sample earned less than $15,000 per year at the time of the interview and 65% earned less than $10,000 per year. Nine percent of the Jewish American participants earned more than $15,000 per year while none of the African

American respondents exceeded that level. In terms of marital status, 86% of the sample was not married and 53% was widowed. However, 29% of the African American group was maritally separated including separation at the time of widowhood compared with only 3% of the Jewish American group. The two groups did not differ on other demographic factors except for religious affiliation and participation.

Patterns in synagogue/church attendance contrasted sharply. Three percent of Jewish American respondents attended synagogue weekly or more, while 51% of African Americans attended religious activities weekly or more. Fifty-nine percent of Jewish American respondents never attended synagogue; 15% of African Americans never attended church. The largest religious affiliation components of the total sample included 31% Baptist and 56% affiliated with the Jewish faith. Forty-one percent of Jewish Americans considered themselves to be secular Jews, identifying with the Jewish culture but not the faith tradition. Twelve diverse faiths were represented, including African Methodist Episcopal (AME), Catholic, and Buddhist.

Life Challenges

How did these groups of older adults conceptualize the life challenges they had encountered? Four general categories of life challenge themes emerged from narrative responses to form an organizing framework. The first and most prevalent theme was personal events/relationship challenges, followed by historical societal challenges, environmental challenges, and personal characteristics challenges. These broad themes are listed in Table 1.

Personal Events/Relationship Challenges. This first category included four subthemes. These were, in order of prevalence: (1) death; (2) health; (3) marital relationships; and (4) family relationships. The death of family and significant friends and coping with subsequent bereavement were identified by 76% of the sample with no ethnic variation. Within these losses, the death of a spouse, a parent, a sibling, or a child was particularly difficult to face. "I lost a daughter to cancer at age 47. That was the hardest thing," reported one Jewish American. As might be expected with an older adult population, health was the second most prevalent life challenge identified by 44% of the sample. In this relatively healthy independent living sample, perceived health differences were not significant across the two groups. An African American male declared, "When I came down with this stroke, I couldn't die, but I wished to. I wouldn't lie and say I wanted to and just didn't. I could not commit suicide, so I thought I might as well

TABLE 1. Life Challenge Summary

	SAMPLE					
	Jewish American		African American		Total	
	No.	%	No.	%	No.	%
Personal Events/Relationships Challenges						
Death: spouse, child, family member, parent	26	(76)	31	(76)	57	(76)
Health: general health problem, cancer, CVA, surgery	15	(44)	18	(44)	33	(44)
Marital Issues: marital problems, divorce, separation	14	(41)	11	(27)	25	(33)
Family Relationship and Parental Role Problems: family of origin, raised child alone	8	(24)	15	(37)	23	(31)
Historical/Societal Challenges						
World War II, Great Depression, Emigration, Discrimination	11	(33)	-	-	11	(15)
Environmental Challenges						
Lack of money, landlord kicked out, male friend stole, etc.	2	(6)	4	(10)	6	(8)
Personal Characteristics Challenges						
Addiction, Alcoholism, Disorganization	3	(9)	-	-	3	(4)
TOTAL	79	-	79	-	158	-

Notes. Jewish American: n = 34, African American: n = 41, Total: N = 75
Total numbers are greater than 75 since as many as three life challenges may have been identified per respondent.
Cumulative percents are > than 100 since more than one problem may have been identified.

live." A Jewish American woman explained, "I went from being healthy to having all kinds of health problems. I have Parkinson's disease and swelling in my feet. I try to be strong, but it's very difficult."

Marital difficulty was another pervasive problem. While 41% of Jewish Americans had marital problems, just over one quarter of African Americans reported these. Respondents described contending with physically abusive and/or alcoholic spouses, lack of respect in the marriage, and abandonment. Divorce and separation were frequent outcomes of these situations, but ongoing commitment was often described by African American respondents alone. As one woman related, "We separated but we're not divorced. He is sick and he lives alone and he has colon cancer. I go over there and do just about everything for him when he's really down." Family relationship problems were also identified. Thirty-seven percent of African American study participants experienced these role strains, but only 24% of Jewish American participants agreed. An African American woman related,

I had a stepmother and I ran away from home. My sister and I both ran away. That particular time when we came along they wasn't called streets. You would meet guys and that's part of life. There never stops being older men that like younger women. They didn't have AIDS then, you know. The police found us and they put us in a home.

Some respondents raised the children of relatives or endured complex relationships with their own offspring, in a few cases dealing with problems such as drug abuse.

Historical/Societal Challenges. This category included historical events that particularly marked this cohort of older adults such as World War II and the Great Depression. This theme reflected the most startling difference between the two groups. No African Americans cited these challenges while one third of Jewish American respondents described experiences in this category.

Discrimination was identified by two Jewish American respondents who were each raised in the only Jewish family in a small town. Although it was also pervasive in the lives of older African American respondents, one of whom wrote to Eleanor Roosevelt about her difficulty finding work and subsequently benefitted from Roosevelt's personal intervention, it was not seen as separate from the interwoven fabric of existence. It was something expected. Any imagination for how life could be different had been effectively eliminated for this cohort of aging older adults who lived with the consequences of unequal treatment, especially in jobs and housing.

Environmental Challenges. This category consisted of episodes like financial difficulties due to limited employment opportunity and being a victim of theft. "There were times I didn't have money, didn't have enough food to eat," acknowledged an African American woman. "Once I had money and a friend, but my friend only wanted my money. I couldn't see that," recounted a Jewish American woman. Tales of betrayal and local injustice marked this grouping, representing 6% of Jewish Americans and 10% of African Americans.

Personal Characteristics Challenges. Internal traits and personal issues characterized problems in this category. Among these challenges were drug addiction, alcoholism, and mental illness. This latter category was the least frequently reported and was reported only by Jewish Americans. It is possible that there were more study participants who experienced similar personal problems, however, this category was also the least socially acceptable one. Respondents would have had to have a strong sense of self-acceptance to reveal these personal "flaws" even in a confidential study. This also may reflect a bias in the sample. Perhaps individuals who were experiencing problems related to personal traits were less likely to agree to participate in a study promoted as investigating how older adults cope with life challenges.

Response Mechanisms

From the data collected about coping with the challenges described previously, four themes emerged (Table 2). These themes, according to prevalence, comprised: (1) social resources; (2) religious resources; (3) personal resources; and (4) idiosyncratic or avoidant coping styles.

Social Resources. Social resources were frequently cited by both groups of older adults (62% of Jewish Americans and 68% of African Americans). Family was viewed as a primary support. A 90-year-old African American woman attributed her sense of well-being to her family, ". . . I have a lot to be grateful for. A lot of it comes from family." Another African American woman indicated that when her husband abandoned her with three small children, her brother came to her aid financially. Family provided concrete assistance such as housing and

TABLE 2. Response Summary

| | SAMPLE | | | | | |
| | Jewish American | | African American | | Total | |
	No.	%	No.	%	No.	%
Social Resources Job, friends, family, community activities	21	(62)	28	(68)	49	(65)
Religious Resources Church community; prayer; resources given by God; Bible/Religion/ Faith	1	(3)	34	(83)	35	(47)
Personal Resources Depended on self; became strong; accepted; Volunteered self for others; used humor; maintained commitment; fulfilled role	22	(73)	13	(32)	35	(47)
Idiosyncratic or Avoidant Styles Trusted doctors; cried; looked to the future; covered up feelings; didn't cope	5	(15)	6	(15)	11	(15)
TOTAL	49	-	81	-	130	-

Notes. Jewish American: n = 34, African American: n = 41, Total: N = 75.
Number may be greater than 75 since more than one response may have been identified.
Cumulative percents are > than 100 since more than one response may have been identified.

funds for siblings who immigrated or migrated north. Family also provided emotional support when respondents were diagnosed with illness.

Friends, too, provided many forms of assistance. Sometimes they listened, providing a sympathetic posture and even guidance or validation. Friends assisted with concrete services like transportation for grocery shopping. One African American man lost his son in a drive-by shooting, his niece in a murder, and his mother to illness within a six-week time frame. "My job kept me going. It was like a little family–everybody had some kind of problems. Everybody just helped each other out through their crisis." In one case a friend shoveled the driveway so one Jewish American respondent could attend her husband's funeral, an act still remembered and appreciated.

Religious Resources. The most striking contrast in coping responses between the two groups was in this area: 3% of Jewish Americans identified use of religious resources versus 83% of African Americans. Relying on one's relationship with God or a Transcendent Force was nominated as a strength by 15 individuals. "I'm helpless without God. That is where my help comes from. I think my relationship with God helps me solve problems," appraised one African American woman. Another affirmed, "You always involve the Lord. You always do that in a crisis."

Closely linked with reliance on a God-relationship was the use of prayer, cited by nine individuals, eight of them African American. One 84-year-old African American woman in poor health reported,

> One thing I believe in is giving all of my trouble to the Lord. In the situation I'm going through, I pray the Lord and ask Him to take me through it. And He can. Any situation. He's able and He has.

Prayer can be impromptu and impulsive (in a critical event) or intentional and sustained (when faced with an ongoing stressor). It is one means of proactively responding to life challenge. Two African American individuals indicated they had little functional capacity to leave the building where they resided to attend church, but prayer was something they could do anywhere, anytime.

Participating in a church or synagogue community with support from others who share a similar life philosophy was identified as an asset by seven individuals (two of whom were Jewish Americans). Rabbis and pastors offered comfort in times of loss by performing tradition-based rituals. A few African American respondents indicated that activities offered through the church gave them assurance that their children would be exposed to positive influences.

Finally, use of the Bible, religion broadly conceived, and faith were named as sources of support. The Bible offered respondents moral guidance, historical lessons, and comfort. One African American participant explained, "The Bible lifts you up and will enlighten you when you're down." Religion also offered principles to live by that informed a response to problems. A female African American minister of a storefront church proclaimed,

> Whatever we learn today, we shouldn't have to be challenged by tomorrow. I had that lesson already. If I failed, then I got to take it over. If you don't want to take it over, do all you can not to fail the lesson of the day. I believe in this. God didn't send me here unequipped. I came fully equipped for whatever demand the world makes of me.

A Jewish American woman experienced faith in specific religious terms, but she also speculated that any form of faith offers merit. She noted, "We make too much of an issue out of denominations and that's not important. The important thing is, we are true believers. Everybody believes in something: It might be Mohammed, it might be the mighty I Am." Belief in something greater than the self was, she thought, a universal means of overcoming adversity.

Personal Resources. Personal resources represented another prominent theme echoed by 73% of Jewish American and 32% of African American respondents. One 76-year-old Jewish American woman spent a decade as a caretaker for her ill mother while also maintaining a position of administrative authority at work. She fulfilled her role as a dutiful daughter, which brought her satisfaction. A second Jewish American woman revealed, "That was a hard time. But somehow or other you cope. I don't know what it is, but you cope. My own hardiness got me through." A third Jewish American who lost her family in World War II affirmed, "I relied on myself. I'm a strong person. I'm a survivor. My peasant heritage has made me strong."

An African American woman dreamed of attending college. Because of limited family finances, only her younger brother was able to attend. Her answer was to enrich her life through reading and to create educational opportunities for her own children. Developing a sense of humor to make others feel comfortable in the presence of his disabled body was one African American man's response.

Idiosyncratic and Avoidant Styles. The final category comprising idiosyncratic and avoidant coping styles was used by an equal proportion

(15%) of each group. One coping style included individuals with health problems who decided that trusting their doctors was a way to control fear of an uncertain medical outcome. Other responses included use of tears to release tension. "What did I do? I cried." One Jewish woman who lost a daughter to cancer 20 years earlier commented, "I never did cope. I never adjusted." A second Jewish American reported a cognitive shift: "There comes a time when you say, 'I'm happy now.' You go along and all of a sudden you realize that you are happy. That's what happened to me."

A Hierarchy of Coping

Analysis of the life challenge categories by individual was conducted to determine if certain types of life challenges elicited certain types of response. For instance, would individuals who identified bereavement issues be more likely to use social or religious resources (Table 3).

TABLE 3. Hierarchy of Coping Responses

Personal Events/ Relationships	Jewish American Coping Style by Percent			African American Coping Style by Percent			Both
	Religious	Social	Personal	Religious	Social	Personal	Total
Death: spouse, child, family member, parent	3	21	24	27	22	12	55
Health: general health problem, cancer, CVA, surgery	3	18	21	25	17	15	49
Family Relationship and Parental Role Problems: family of origin, raised child alone	-	6	18	25	10	5	33
Marital Issues: marital problems, divorce, separation	-	6	9	10	7	2	17
Historical Societal Challenges	-	6	8	-	-	-	15

Notes. African American: N = 41, Jewish American: N = 34, Total: N = 75
Not all individuals identified each area as a life challenge they had experienced. Of those that did, some individuals used more than one coping style. Percents shown are summed responses for first, second, and third choices in coping style. A weighted score was also calculated, but there was no difference in hierarchical order of coping responses. All percents are of the total N of 75.

Across all of the Personal Events/Relationships domains–death, health, marriage, and family relationships–to which the largest numbers of respondents subscribed, a pattern emerged that is consistent by race. African American respondents were most likely to use religious resources, followed by social resources and finally personal resources. Jewish American respondents were most likely to report using personal resources, followed by social resources and finally religious resources as a distant third. This pattern held for Historical/Societal Challenges which only Jewish respondents endorsed. There was insufficient data in the last two categories to make a valid comparison, though the pattern was similar. The two groups had distinctly different hierarchies of coping styles.

DISCUSSION AND CONCLUSIONS

Life challenges were experienced in contrasting ways across the two groups of study participants. Both groups identified bereavement challenges and health issues as major difficulties, but Jewish Americans more commonly identified marital relationships as concerns while family relationship problems (apart from marital) were more frequently described by African American respondents. These results are illustrative of cultural differences regarding the trajectories of marriage and family. While nearly one half of Jewish Americans in this sample were widows/widowers, nearly 30% of African Americans in this study were maritally separated, not widowed. This is consistent with research that shows African American women spend less of their lives married than do European American women, are less likely to be married in old age, and experience a lower financial penalty for ending a marriage (Willson, 2003; Cherlin, 1992). Also, the extended kin network was very important to the well-being of African American respondents. There was an expectation that family support would be present. When this wasn't available or the connection was ruptured, the loss was identified as a great stressor.

Limited economic opportunity, factors like unemployment and employment in low-wage sectors, was more likely to affect older African Americans in this study. Many women in the African American group had worked in the "domestics" industry as maids or cooks, often with no social security taken out of paychecks. While Jewish Americans were approximately equal to African American respondents in current income, it was clear that there were differences in lifelong earning patterns. Some of the former had received very high incomes in previous periods; literally, they had made and lost fortunes. As a result, expectations of where they would be financially at this stage in their lives may have differed strongly from their reality. Financial security for Jewish American women was more closely tied to marriage. While income was often cited as a stressor in narratives, it was not generally identified as a major life challenge.

What was missing in the life challenge categories for African Americans compared to Jewish Americans was noteworthy. None of the African American respondents identified the ways historical events indelibly marked their generation. Absent was identification of discrimination practices or the hardships of World War II, though both were present in the stories they told. These events and conditions formed the broad overlay of their lives and were not extracted as particular hardships, perhaps because they could imagine life to be no different. If true, this stands as a broad indictment of racism and discrimination in the United States cultural context.

Respondents in this study did not view major life challenge as being the consequence of their individual action to a large extent, but rather a consequence of environmental press. The outcomes of many life challenges lay beyond their ability to completely control. However, respondents enjoyed an extensive array of choice in their response opportunities. It is likely that the particular responses set in motion were a function of dispositional (personal) characteristics combined with environmental possibilities; however, dispositional characteristics were not addressed in this study to the same extent as contextual factors. While social supports were widely held to be a major resource across both groups, only African American respondents conspicuously listed religious resources as a major benefit. Personal resources were more likely to be mentioned by Jewish Americans than African Americans. These were the areas of greatest difference in coping responses across the groups.

African American respondents relied on religious faith or religious community. Jewish American respondents relied on themselves and their own initiative first. The power of the type of problem was less salient than the power of race/ethnicity. In other words, no matter what the problem was, individuals tended to cope with it using the same general philosophical approach. If religion was the primary coping model, it was applied equally to issues of bereavement, health, etc. If personal initiative was the primary approach, then that was applied no matter which life challenge was encountered.

This hierarchy of coping styles that emerged from the data parallels a similar formulation advanced by Cantor in regard to social support

(Cantor, Brennan, & Sainz, 1994; Messeri, Silverstein, & Litwak, 1993). She found that the choice of caregivers for an older adult followed an ordered preference based on the primacy of the relationship– whether the caregiver was spouse, other relative, or friend. She named this the hierarchical-compensatory model. Likewise in this study, respondents provided first and sometimes second and third choices about how they managed a particular life challenge, but there was a clear preference for coping style by race/ethnicity.

There are several explanations for this hierarchy of coping resources. First, the church has provided a cultural as well as a religious center in the African American community. Since the last century, it has served as a haven and a place of empowerment. According to Gilkes (1998), the black church has held or increased membership in contrast to American mainline denominations, which have decreased. It has sought to foster social justice and economic equity. Furthermore, the African American church was perceived as a source of connection, a place of class reintegration and solidarity as well as a mechanism for effective advocacy. In essence it has functioned as a therapeutic community even for those unable to attend. While associations with the temple or synagogue may be weak for Jewish Americans (less than 13% of Jews attend regularly [Roof & McKinney, 1987]), the sense of ethnic identity remains strong, as it did for Jewish Americans in this study. They did not attend synagogue in large numbers and did not use religious resources, but they did retain a sense of cultural affiliation that was evident through the narratives.

Secondly, personal coping was a style in which Jewish Americans and some African Americans took great pride. Across the life course, two thirds of Jewish American and one third of African American individuals reported that they learned to rely on themselves, adjust, and manage. There was a sense of not giving up, of just going on with life in difficult circumstances. Dispositional factors such as self-efficacy (Bandura, 1982), hardiness (Kobasa, Maddi, & Kahn, 1982) and an internal locus of control (Lefcourt, 1992) are particularly important as coping resources. This attitude of active self-reliance was particularly strong in the former group, based on cultural congruence and the value of identity as a people that helped Jewish Americans to survive discriminatory practices. Thirdly, both groups subscribed to the value of enlisting the support of family and friends, consistent with the large body of literature on social support that indicates that emotional support boosts feelings of self-esteem and self-confidence (Carpenter & Scott, 1992; Lubben, 1988; Messeri, Silverstein, & Litwak, 1993).

The hierarchy of coping styles does coincide with Lazarus and Folkman's model of emotion-focused and problem-focused coping. While religious coping contains some active components such as participation in religious ritual, it also helps individuals regulate emotional adjustment to life challenges that they may not be able to change. Personal coping as described by respondents in this study is typically an action-based or problem-focused approach where individuals design strategies to alter the situation. Social coping can have aspects of both styles of coping dependent on the type of social support engaged, whether emotional or concrete.

Limitations

This study was limited because it used a purposive sample, so results are not generalizable. It is difficult to know how representative the results may be, however, the large number of in-depth interviews resulted in a rich source of information about urban-dwelling low-income minority populations. Results suggest that Jewish and African American older adults approach stressors using one or two styles that have been useful to them in the past. Although there was not enough data to confirm this pattern beyond the categories of personal events/processes and historical/societal challenges, the small numbers in the remaining two categories did not refute this trend.

A second limitation concerns memory. Since respondents were asked to identify the most salient life challenges they had experienced looking at their lives retrospectively, there is potential for confounding due to issues of memory retrieval that tend to promote events from childhood and more recent events over those occurring in middle age. Longitudinal research studies are needed to further discern whether older adults use different resources at different points in their lives or find the same ones to be effective throughout. This information can assist mental health practitioners to focus on prior client strengths and suggest ways these can be accessed to meet present needs. A third limitation was that fewer men resided in the housing sites, and therefore men were poorly represented in this qualitative study. Since the life expectancy for men continues to rise, it is important to know specifically how they adapt to the challenges of later life and what supports they especially will require.

Implications

Implications for practice are especially important in relation to client assessment. They include orienting practitioners to the types of challenges African American and Jewish American older adults have faced that will influence how they manage new challenges of aging. Prior mastery over life challenge can help people flourish and exhibit resilience in new circumstances. It is valuable for social workers and other mental health practitioners to understand how diverse groups of ethnic elders appraise life challenges, so that they can be adequately supported. One of these challenges includes a subtext of marginalization that may have meaning for the coping response or the repertoire of responses these clients will find most valuable.

A hierarchy of coping responses suggests social resources can be strengthened in the form of helping both groups of older adults access networks of family and friends. For African Americans particularly, religious resources can be reinforced or referrals can be made to clergy and/or church communities. Jewish Americans can be reminded, where appropriate, of the ways they have previously and successfully drawn on their own strengths. The primary coping style identified can be shaped to meet current circumstances. Although clients' individual preferences may be unique and should always be sought, building an understanding of the types of resources that Jewish American and African American older adults typically use in dealing with difficult challenges will help mental health professionals be more efficient in collaborating on treatment decisions with these clients.

REFERENCES

Bandura, A. (1982). Self-efficacy mechanism in human agency. *American Psychologist, 37*, 122-147.

Billings, A.G., & Moos, R.H. (1981). The role of coping responses and social resources in attenuating the impact of stressful life events. *Journal of Behavioral Medicine, 4,* 139-157.

Binstock, R., & George, L. (1990). *Race, ethnicity and aging: Conceptual and methodological issues.* Boston, MA: Academic Press.

Bjorck, J.P., & Cohen, L.H. (1993). Coping with threats, losses, and challenges. *Journal of Social and Clinical Psychology, 12,* 36-72.

Bowles, J., Brooks, T., Hayes-Reams, P., Butts, T., Myers, H., Allen, W., & Kington, R. (2000). Frailty, family, and church support among urban African-American elderly. *Journal of Health Care for the Poor and Underserved, 11*(1), 87-99.

Cantor, M.H., Brennan, M., & Sainz, A. (1994). The importance of ethnicity in the social support systems of older New Yorkers: A longitudinal perspective. *Journal of Gerontological Social Work, 22*(3-4), 95-128.

Carpenter, B.N., & Scott, S.M. (1992). Interpersonal aspects of coping. In B.N. Carpenter (Ed.), *Personal coping: Theory research, and application* (pp. 93-109). New York: Praeger.

Cherlin, A.J. (1992). *Marriage, divorce, remarriage.* Cambridge, MA: Harvard University Press.

Ellison, C.G., & Taylor, R.J. (1996). Turning to prayer: Social and situational antecedents of religious coping among African Americans. *Review of Religious Research, 38*, 111-131.

Fiske, S. (1993). Controlling other people: The impact of power on stereotyping. *American Psychologist* (June), 621-628.

Gilkes, C.T. (1998). Plenty good room: Adaptation in a changing black church. In W.C. Roof (Ed.), *America and religions in the 21st century, the annals of the American academy of political and social science, 558*, 101-121.

Glaser, B.G., & Strauss, A.L. (1967). *The discovery of grounded theory: Strategies for qualitative research.* New York: Aldine de Gruyter.

Gottlieb, B.H. (1997). *Coping with chronic stress.* New York: Plenum Press.

Heppner P.P., & Petersen, C.H. (1982). The development and implications of a personal problem-solving inventory. *Journal of Counseling Psychology, 29*(1), 66-75.

Hooyman, N.R., & Kiyak, H.A. (1999). *Social gerontology: A multidisciplinary perspective.* Boston, MA: Allyn & Bacon.

Hooyman, N.R., & Kiyak, H.A. (2002). *Social gerontology: A multidisciplinary perspective.* Boston, MA: Allyn & Bacon.

Jackson, J., Chatters, L., & Taylor, R. (1993). *Aging in Black America.* Thousand Oaks, CA: Sage.

Jones, F., & Kinman, G. (2001). Approaches to studying stress. In F. Jones & J. Bright (Eds.), *Stress: Myth, theory and research* (pp. 17-45). New York: Prentice Hall.

Kahana, E., Kahana, B., Kercher, K., King, C., Lovegreen, L., & Chirayath, H. (1999). Evaluating a model of successful aging for urban African American and White elderly. In M.L. Wylke & A.B. Ford (Eds.), *Serving minority elders in the 21st century* (pp. 287-322). New York: Springer.

Kahana, E., Redmond, C., Hill, G., Kercher, K., Kahana, B., Johnson, J.R., & Young, R.F. (1995). The effects of stress, vulnerability, and appraisals on the psychological well being of the elderly. *Research on Aging, 17*(4), 459-489.

Kobasa, S.C., Maddi, S.R., & Kahn, S. (1982). Hardiness and health: A prospective study. *Journal of Personality and Social Psychology, 42*, 168-172.

Koenig, H.G. (1995). Commentary: Religion as cognitive schema. *The International Journal for the Psychology of Religion, 5*(1), 31-37.

Koenig, H.G., McCullough, M.E., & Larson, D.B. (2001). *Handbook of religion and health.* Oxford: Oxford University Press.

Lazarus, R.S., & Folkman, S. (1984). *Stress, appraisal, and coping.* New York: Springer Publishing Company.

Lazarus, R.S., & Folkman, S. (1989). *Manual for the hassles and uplifts scale.* Palo Alto, CA: Consulting Psychologists Press.

Lefcourt, H.M. (1992). Perceived control, personal effectiveness, and emotional states. In B.N. Carpenter (Ed.), *Personal coping: Theory research, and application* (pp. 111-131). New York: Praeger.

Lubben, J.E. (1988). Assessing social networks among elderly populations. *Family and Community Health, 11*(3), 42-52.

McInnis-Dittrich, K. (2002). *Social work with elders.* Boston: Allyn & Bacon.

Messeri, P., Silverstein, M., & Litwak, E. (1993). Choosing optimal support groups: A review and reformulation. *Journal of Health and Social Behavior, 34*(June), 122-137.

Miley, K.K., O'Melia, M., & DuBois, B. (2001). *Generalist social work practice: An empowering approach* (3rd ed.). Boston: Allyn & Bacon.

Myerhoff, B. (1992). Life not death in Venice. In M. Kaminsky (Ed.), *Remembered lives: The work of ritual, storytelling, and growing older* (pp. 257-276). Ann Arbor, MI: University of Michigan Press.

Nelson-Becker, H.B. (1999). Spiritual and religious problem-solving in older adults: Mechanisms for managing life challenge (Doctoral Dissertation, The University of Chicago, 1999). *Dissertation Abstracts International,* 60-08, 253 p.

Neugarten, G.L., Havighurst, R.J., & Tobin, S.S. (1961). The measurement of life satisfaction. *Journal of Gerontology, 16,* 134-143.

Roof, W.C., & McKinney, W. (1987*). American mainline religion: Its changing shape and future.* New Brunswick: Rutgers University Press.

Snyder, C.R. (2001). *Coping with stress: Effective people and processes.* Oxford: University Press.

Willson, A.E. (2003). Race and women's income trajectories: Employment, marriage, and income security over the life course. *Social Problems, 50* (1), 87-110.

Yesavage, J.A., Brink, T.L., Rose, T.L., & Leirer, V.O. (1983). Development and validation of a geriatric depression screening scale. A preliminary report. *Journal of Psychiatric Research, 17,* 37-49.

Zeidner, M., & Endler, N.S. (Eds.) (1996). *Handbook of coping.* New York: John Wiley & Sons, Inc.

Depression and Religiosity
in African American
and White Community-Dwelling
Older Adults

Lucinda Lee Roff
David L. Klemmack
Michael Parker
Harold G. Koenig
Martha Crowther
Patricia S. Baker
Richard M. Allman

Lucinda Lee Roff, PhD, David L. Klemmack, PhD, Michael Parker, DSW, and Martha Crowther, PhD, are all affiliated with the University of Alabama. Harold G. Koenig, MD, is affiliated with the Duke University Medical Center. Patricia S. Baker, PhD, is affiliated with The University of Alabama at Birmingham (UAB). Richard M. Allman, MD, is affiliated with the University of Alabama at Birmingham (UAB) and the Birmingham/Atlanta VA Geriatric Research, Education and Clinical Center.

Address correspondence to: Lucinda Lee Roff, University of Alabama, Box 870314, Tuscaloosa, AL 35487.

This research was funded by the National Institute on Aging (NIA Grant AG150602) and the AARP/Andrus Foundation. Though the views expressed in this article are the exclusive opinions of its authors, the authors gratefully acknowledge the assistance of the John A. Hartford Foundation's Geriatric Social Work Faculty Scholars Program.

[Haworth co-indexing entry note]: "Depression and Religiosity in African American and White Community-Dwelling Older Adults." Roff, Lucinda Lee et al. Co-published simultaneously in *Journal of Human Behavior in the Social Environment* (The Haworth Social Work Practice Press, an imprint of The Haworth Press, Inc.) Vol. 10, No. 1, 2004, pp. 175-189; and: *Diversity and Aging in the Social Environment* (eds: Sherry M. Cummings, and Colleen Galambos) The Haworth Social Work Practice Press, an imprint of The Haworth Press, Inc., 2004, pp. 175-189. Single or multiple copies of this article are available for a fee from The Haworth Document Delivery Service [1-800-HAWORTH, 9:00 a.m. - 5:00 p.m. (EST). E-mail address: docdelivery@haworthpress.com].

175

SUMMARY. This research examined the extent to which religiosity was predictive of level of depression, even after controlling for race, gender, social support, income sufficiency, and physical health. Data were collected using in-home interviews conducted from 1999 to 2001 with 1,000 adults age 65 to 106. Subjects were recruited from a stratified, random sample of Medicare beneficiaries age 65 and older in five central Alabama counties (three rural and two urban). The sample was stratified by county, race, and sex and included balanced numbers of African American males and females and White males and females. Highly religious persons had lower levels of depression, even when controlling for other known covariates, $\beta = -.16$, $t(972)$ $p < .001$. Females reported higher levels of depression, $\beta = .07$, $t(972)$ $p < .05$. Although race was unrelated to depression in the model including gender and religiosity only, African Americans reported fewer symptoms of depression than did Whites when social support, income sufficiency, and physical health were added to the model, $\beta = -.08$, $t(972)$ $p < .01$. Results suggest the importance of health and social service professionals' drawing upon older adults' positive spirituality in professional interventions to prevent and treat depression. *[Article copies available for a fee from The Haworth Document Delivery Service: 1-800-HAWORTH. E-mail address: <docdelivery@haworthpress.com> Website: <http://www.HaworthPress.com> © 2004 by The Haworth Press, Inc. All rights reserved.]*

KEYWORDS. Older adults, elderly, depression, religiosity, diversity, gender, race, African Americans, social support, health, socioeconomic status

INTRODUCTION

The focus of this paper is the relationship between religiosity and symptoms of depression among Southern, community-dwelling older persons who are diverse by race and by gender. We consider the extent to which their religiosity is predictive of their level of depression even after their race, their gender, and a number of resource factors (physical health, financial resources, and social support) are controlled.

Depression is a mental health problem affecting significant proportions of African American and White male and female elders (Blazer, Landerman, Hays, Simonsick, & Saunders, 1998; Blazer, Hughes, & George, 1987; Kennedy et al., 1989; Lebowitz et al., 1997). Recent estimates (Alexopoulus, 1997; Gallo & Lebowitz, 1999) indicate that from eight to 20% of community dwelling elders experience depression, as do 17%-35% of primary care patients (Gurland, Cross, & Katz, 1996). Similarly Lebowitz et al. (1997) report that subsyndromal depressions affect 13-27% of community-dwelling older adults and up to 50% of those who are medically ill and nursing home residents. By 2050, the population age 65 and older will increase to 20% of the total U.S. population, with the White population doubling and the African American elderly population quadrupling (U.S. Bureau of the Census, 2000). Depression among older adults has been termed a major "public health problem" to which health and social service professionals should attend in order to "minimize suffering, improve overall functioning and quality of life, and limit inappropriate use of health care resources" (Lebowitz et al., 1997, p. 1186). Social workers will increasingly find themselves working with older adults who experience significant depressive symptoms in both inpatient and community-based settings. Thus, an in-depth understanding of environmental and psycho- social factors associated with depression in later life among older adults is important.

Increasing attention has been focused in recent years on the relationship between religious/spiritual belief and practice, and health and mental health outcomes (George, 2002; Idler, 2002; Koenig, McCullough, & Larson, 2001; Larson et al., 1992). A growing body of scientific research is finding positive relationships between religious activity and belief and mental health, including studies that have shown that religious persons report less depression. Koenig et al.'s (2001) review of cross-sectional studies linking organized religious activity with depression found that in more than 85%, participation in organized religion was associated with lower depression. Religious coping was inversely related to depression among geriatric hospitalized men (Koenig et al., 1992) and to cognitive but not somatic symptoms of depression in a follow-up study (Koenig et al., 1995). Among community-dwelling elders with cancer, religious activity was related to fewer depressive symptoms, with the effects stronger for African Americans than for Whites (Musick, Koenig, Hays, & Cohen, 1998). There is some evidence that non-organizational and intrinsic religiosity are also associated with lower levels of depression (Kendler, Gardner, & Prescott, 1997).

At the same time social workers are placing renewed emphasis on the importance of religiosity/spirituality in the lives of the people they serve and are recommending that spiritual assessments become regular components of psychosocial assessments (Canda & Furman, 1999; Martin &

Martin, 2002). Thus, the relationship between religious/spiritual dimensions of older persons' lives and their experiences of depression is an important topic for social work practitioners.

This research addresses possible effects of respondents' gender and race on the relationship between religiosity and depression for two reasons. First, there are continuing questions about whether the contemporary mental health system appropriately serves older women and African Americans (Mays, 1985; Mays, Caldwell, & Jackson, 1996), and it is thus important to focus on these vulnerable groups. Second, there is research evidence to indicate there are differential rates of depression by race and gender among older adults. Thus, it is important to understand whether any relationship found between religiosity and depression might be better accounted for by gender or race.

A considerable body of research literature shows that females are more likely to report depression in later life than are males (Hybels, Blazer, & Pieper, 2001; Mulsant & Ganguli, 1999; Musick, Blazer, & Hays, 2000; Roberts, Kaplan, Shema, & Strawbridge, 1997). There is also evidence to suggest that older females experience depression somewhat differently than males (Kockler & Heun, 2002). Brown, Milburn, and Gary (1992), however, found no difference in depression between males and females in their sample of community-based African American elders.

The literature comparing the prevalence of depression symptoms among older African Americans and Whites shows mixed results (Blazer et al., 1998; Callahan & Wolinsky, 1994; Smallegan, 1989; Eaton & Kessler, 1981; Fiscella & Franks, 1997; Gallo, Cooper-Patrick, & Lesikar, 1998), with some studies finding lower symptomatology among African Americans and others finding higher symptomatology. Cochran, Brown and McGregor (1999) found higher levels of depressive symptoms among African American women age 55-61 than among White women. Gallo et al. (1998) found that older African Americans reported dysphoria less frequently than Whites. In studies that focused solely on African Americans, Bazargan and Hamm-Baugh (1995) found depression greatest among African Americans with more financial difficulties and less social support, and Okwumabua, Baker, Wong, and Pilgram (1997) found that medical illness and social network were important predictors of depressive symptoms in African Americans.

Among the environmental and psychosocial resource factors that have received the most theoretical and research attention in relation to depression are those related to physical health, financial resources, and social support. Persons who are in poorer physical health tend to be more depressed than those who are in better physical health (Adams, 2001; Hybels et al., 2001; Koenig et al., 1997a; Mulsant & Ganguli, 1999; Roberts et al., 1997). Persons with less adequate incomes are more likely to be depressed than are those with more adequate incomes (Adams, 2001; Mitchell, Mathews, & Yesavage 1993; Roberts et al., 1997). Also, persons who report higher levels of social support tend to be less depressed (Adams, 2001; Hybels et al., 2001; Koenig et al., 1997; Mitchell et al., 1993). Similarly, Hays et al. (1998) found that having a confidant was associated with positive affect for community-dwelling elders. We were thus interested in whether any relationship found between religiosity and depression could be attributable to physical health, financial resources or social support.

Within this context, this study posed three questions:

1. Did highly religious older adults report fewer symptoms of depression than those who were not highly religious?
2. Did adding race and gender to the prediction model change any relationship previously found between religiosity and depression?
3. Did adding resource variables (social support, income sufficiency, physical health) to the model change the relationships previously found between religiosity and depression?

METHODS

Sample

Data for this study were collected from in-home interviews conducted from 1999 to 2001 with 1,000 adults age 65 to 106 recruited from a stratified, random sample of Medicare beneficiaries in five central Alabama counties (three rural and two urban). The sample was stratified by county, race, and sex, with balanced numbers of African American males and females and White males and females. Table 1 presents descriptive statistics for the sample and all study variables.

Measures

The short, 15-item form of the Geriatric Depression Scale was used to assess depression in this study. Scores can range from 0 to 15. When the GDS short form is used as a screening tool, it is recommended that individuals who score six or higher be referred for a more comprehen-

TABLE 1. Summary Statistics for Study Variables (*N* = 979)

Item	*M*	*SD*
Geriatric Depression Scale	2.36	2.33
AIMS 2 Lack of Social Support Subscale	6.08	3.03
Income sufficiency	2.76	0.97
General physical health (PCS12)	39.71	12.97
Age	75.26	6.69
	%	
Female	50%	
African American	50%	
Highly religious	43%	

sive assessment and accurate diagnosis (Yesavage, 2002). Coefficient alpha with these respondents was .73.

The measure of religiosity used in this study was a slightly modified version of the Duke University Religion Index (DUREL) (Koenig, Meador, & Parkerson, 1997b). This five-item measure captures the three major dimensions of religiousness presented by Koenig and Futterman (1995). Respondents who indicated that they attended church at least weekly (organizational religiosity), prayed more than weekly (non-organizational religiosity) and answered "*definitely true of me*" to three statements measuring intrinsic religiosity were defined as highly religious. The three statements measuring intrinsic religiosity (IR) were: "In my life, I experience the presence of the Divine (i.e., God)," "My religious beliefs are really what lie behind my whole approach to life," and "I try hard to carry my religion over into all other dealings in life." Koenig et al. (1997b) selected these items as a measure of IR based on their loadings on the IR factor of a principal components factor analysis of the Hoge 10-item scale of intrinsic religiosity. Coefficient alpha for these three items was .83, suggesting that these items measured a single concept. The religiosity variable was dichotomized into highly religious (i.e., respondents scoring high on organizational, non-organizational, and intrinsic religiosity) and all other respondents.

Two measures of diversity, gender and race, were added to the regression equation. Gender and race were presented in the Medicare beneficiary list and confirmed by the interviewer.

Social support was measured using the social support subscale of the Arthritis Impact Measure (AIMS 2) (Ren, Kazis, & Meenan, 1999). This subscale ranges from 4 to 20 with a higher score representing lower social support. Coefficient alpha with these respondents was .79. Income sufficiency was measured by a single self-report item on a scale ranging from 1 (is not enough to make ends meet) to 4 (allows you to do more or less what you want). The measure of physical health was the 12-item physical health subscale (PCS-12) of the SF-12 (Ware, Kosinski, & Keller, 1995), which ranged from 0 (poor health) to 100 (excellent health). The SF-12 is a 12 item, commercially available test of physical health status derived from the Medical Outcomes Study 36-Item Short-Form Health Survey (Ware, Kosinski, & Keller, 1996). Two-week test-retest correlations for the instrument ranged from 0.76 to 0.89, and the median relative validity estimates ranged from 0.43 (musculoskeletal symptom cluster) to 0.77 (comorbid conditions, Ware et al., 1996).

Analysis

We used hierarchical regression to analyze the data. In the first stage we used religiosity to predict depression. In the second stage, we introduced race and sex as controls to determine if they eliminated the relationship between religiosity and depression. In the third and final stage we further controlled for resource variables known to be related to depression (social support, income adequacy, and physical health).

RESULTS

All analyses were restricted to the 979 subjects (of 1,000 in the sample) for whom we had complete information on all of the study variables. Subjects ranged in age from 65 to 106, with 51.5% (N = 505) being less than 75 and 11.1% (N = 109) being 85 or older (see Table 1). The sample was divided approximately equally by gender (490 males and 489 females), race (489 Whites and 490 African Americans), and place of residence (471 urban and 508 rural). Approximately one fifth of the respondents (20.2% or 198) had completed six or fewer years of school, 50% (N = 489) had less than a high school education, and 26.2% (N = 257) had completed more than high school. Approximately 29% (N = 281) reported that their income was sufficient to allow them to do "more or less what they wanted," another 27% (N = 266) said their income "kept them comfortable but permitted no luxuries," 35% (N = 345) reported their income was "just enough to get by on," and 9% (N = 87) said their income was "not enough to make ends meet." Slightly over half (N = 495) of the respondents scored four on the measure of social support, indicating they perceived that they "always" had the support of their family and friends. Finally, 42.6% (N = 417) of the respondents scored high on all three dimensions of the customized DUREL, suggesting a high level of religiosity.

On average, respondents reported having slightly more than two of the 15 symptoms ($M = 2.36$, $SD = 2.33$) and 10% (98 of 979) scored six or higher on the GDS (above the cutoff for possible depression). An additional 14.6% reported four or five symptoms, suggesting the possibility of subsyndromal depression. These levels of depression symptoms were similar to those found in other community-based studies of older adults.

There was no statistically significant difference between females and males (10.4% vs. 9.6%) or between African Americans and Whites (11.4% vs. 8.6%) in their likelihood of having a GDS score of six or higher. Highly religious respondents were substantially less likely than respondents who were less religious to have a GDS score of six or higher (5.8% vs. 13.2%, $\chi^2(1) = 14.60$, $p < .001$).

The most common symptoms of depression reported were "preferring to stay home rather than going out and doing new things" and "not feeling full of energy" (see Table 2). These items were included in the six-item WAV (withdrawal, apathy and lack of vigor) scale proposed by Adams (2001) in her analysis of the 36-item long form of the GDS.

Consistent with previous literature (Koenig et al., 2001), older adults who were highly religious had fewer symptoms of depression than did those who were less religious, $\beta = -.20$, $t(977) = -6.44$, $p < .001$. This relationship remained largely unchanged with the introduction of gender and race, $\beta = -.22$, $t(975) = -6.91$, $p < .001$. With the further addition of resource measures to the model there was some attenuation in the relationship between religiosity and depression, $\beta = -.16$, $t(972) = -5.56$, $p < .001$.

When we introduced the diversity measures in the second stage of the analysis, gender but not race, was related to depression, indicating that women were more likely to be depressed than men, $\beta = .09$, $t(975) = 2.95$, $p < .005$. However, when the resource measures were added, race emerged as a predictor, with African Americans having somewhat fewer symptoms of depression than Whites, $\beta = -.08$, $t(972) = -2.76$, $p < .001$, and women continuing to have more symptoms than men, $\beta = .07$, $t(972) = 2.42$, $p < .05$.

Consistent with previous work, physical health and income sufficiency emerged as strong predictors of depression. Older adults who

TABLE 2. Percent Reporting Different Symptoms of Depression on the Geriatric Depression Scale (N = 979)

Item	Percent
Do you prefer to stay at home rather than go out and do new things?	50.8
*Do you feel full of energy?	42.1
Do you often get bored?	24.2
Do you feel you have more problems with memory than most?	18.6
Have you dropped many of your activities and interests?	17.2
Do you think most people are better off than you are?	14.0
Do you often feel helpless?	13.6
Do you feel that your life is empty?	12.5
Do you feel pretty worthless the way you are now?	9.9
Do you feel that your situation is hopeless?	8.4
Are you afraid that something bad is going to happen to you?	7.2
*Are you basically satisfied with your life?	6.7
*Do you feel happy most of the time?	6.1
*Are you in good spirits most of the time?	3.6
*Do you think it is wonderful to be alive now?	1.2

*Item reverse scored so that answering "no" reflects a symptom of depression

were in better physical health had fewer symptoms of depression, $\beta = -.31$, $t(972) = -10.51$, $p < .001$, and those who perceived their incomes to be more sufficient for their needs also had fewer symptoms, $\beta = -.26$, $t(972) = -8.11$, $p < .001$. The magnitude of the relationship of social support to depression was similar to that of religiosity. Respondents with strong social support reported fewer symptoms of depression, $\beta = .14$, $t(972) = 5.09$, $p < .001$.

DISCUSSION

Health and social service personnel working with older adults have a number of goals concerning late life depression. Ideally, they want to prevent its occurrence. Failing that, they seek to identify depression in its early stages and offer intervention so that the condition is treated successfully and does not recur. We discuss the findings of the present study in the context of these goals.

TABLE 3. Hierarchical Regression Analysis for Selected Characteristics on the Geriatric Depression Scale (N = 979)

	Step 1			Step 2			Step 3		
	B	SE B	β	B	SE B	β	B	SE B	β
Religiosity	−.95	.148	−.20***	−1.03	.149	−.22***	−.74	.134	−.16***
Diversity measures									
Gender				0.43	.147	0.09**	0.32	.131	0.07*
Race				0.27	.145	0.06	−.39	.142	−.08**
Resource measures									
Lack of social support							0.11	.021	0.14***
Income sufficiency							−.62	.077	−.26***
Physical health							−.06	.005	−.31***

Note. R² = .04 for Step 1; ΔR² = .01 for Step 2; ΔR² = .21 for Step 3.
*p < .05; ** p < .01; *** p < .001

A major finding of this study was that high religiosity was associated with lower depression scores. The predictive value of religiosity overshadowed that of both race and gender. This suggests the importance of drawing upon clients' religious and spiritual resources in professional interventions (Crowther et al., 2002). Health and social service personnel should routinely conduct spiritual assessments of their older clients. In times of crisis, ill health, or loss it will be important for the health or social service professional to support the highly religious client's religious practice and tradition in efforts to prevent or mitigate depression.

Consistent with previous work, good physical health and income sufficiency predicted the absence of depressive symptoms in this sample, underscoring the importance of all efforts to promote good health and income sufficiency in later life as also ways to help maintain good mental health among older persons.

Social workers who serve African American elders at risk of depression should consider the church as an important partner in their work. Others have found that older African Americans with mental health problems, particularly those who are highly religious, are less likely to use traditional mental health services and look to the church as a primary source of help (Mays et al., 1996). Further, in a recent study of primary care patients, African Americans were three times as likely to view spirituality as important in depression care as were their White counterparts (Cooper, Brown, Vu, Ford, & Powe, 2001). Thus, culturally appropriate, faith-based interventions to help older adults deal with depression could reduce needless suffering for many. The parish nurse model (Solari-Twadell & McDermott, 1999) may be a helpful model for social workers to consult in developing mental health-oriented partnerships with faith-based organizations. Martin and Martin (2002) provide a thoughtful rationale and guidelines for incorporating spirituality into social work interventions with African Americans.

Since older females in general are more likely than older males to be church attenders (Ploch & Hastings, 1994), church-based programs to identify and alleviate depression may be helpful for women of other races as well. Because some 58% of older persons inappropriately believe that depression is a normal consequence of aging (O'Neill, 2002), it is particularly important that clergy and other professionals associated with faith-based programs correct this misinformation.

This study's findings not only suggest some directions about how to go about preventing depression among older adults, they also provide some guidance about efforts to screen and identify older adults at risk for depression so that early interventions can be offered. Depression screening programs for older adults, conducted through faith-based, community-based, or primary care settings, should focus on White women of poorer health and lower income, with lower social support and lower religiosity. On the basis of this study's findings, such persons would be more at risk for presenting symptoms of depression than others. Some of these same characteristics, however, make these individuals particularly difficult to identify for screening and intervention programs. This suggests the possibility of creative outreach programs to reach underdiagnosed and underserved elders.

Activities and interventions in the community aimed at helping older adults remain active and involved may help prevent the onset of symptoms of apathy and withdrawal, particularly in the face of the losses and health declines that are typical of later life. Programs such as those in senior centers, congregate nutrition sites, and church-based activity programs for seniors may serve this function, since attendance at religious services is clearly associated with lower rates of depression among older adults (Idler, 1987; Idler, Kasl, & Hays, 2001; Koenig et al., 2001).

In their efforts to counter depression and contribute to high-quality lives for older persons, health and social service professionals can refer elders at risk of withdrawal to communities of faith and other meaningful opportunities for participation. They can also go a step further by helping to create and support opportunities in local communities where elders can make significant and valued contributions.

REFERENCES

Adams, K.B. (2001). Depressive symptoms, depletion, or developmental change? Withdrawal, apathy, and lack of vigor in the Geriatric Depression Scale. *The Gerontologist, 41*, 768-777.

Alexopoulos, G.S. (1997, November 6). *Epidemiology, nosology and treatment of geriatric depression.* Paper presented at Exploring Opportunities to Advance Mental Health Care for an Aging Population, meeting sponsored by the John A. Hartford Foundation, Rockville, MD.

Bazargan, M., & Hamm-Baugh, V.P. (1995). The relationship between chronic illness and depression in a community of urban black elderly persons. *Journals of Gerontology Series B: Psychological Sciences and Social Sciences, 50*, S-119-S127.

Blazer, D., Hughes, D., & George, L. (1987). The epidemiology of depression in an elderly community population. *The Gerontologist, 27*, 281-287.

Blazer, D.G., Landerman, L.R., Hays, J.C., Simonsick, E.M., & Saunders, W.B. (1998). Symptoms of depression among community-dwelling elderly African-American and White older adults. *Psychological Medicine, 28*, 1311-1320.

Brown, D.R., Milburn, N.G., & Gary, L.E. (1992). Symptoms of depression among older African-Americans: An analysis of gender differences. *The Gerontologist, 32*, 789-795.

Callahan, C., & Wolinsky, F. (1994). Effect of gender and race on the measurement properties of the CES-D in older adults. *Medical Care, 32*, 341-356.

Canda, E.R., & Furman, L.D. (1999). *Spiritual diversity in social work practice: The heart of helping.* New York: The Free Press.

Cochran, D.L., Brown, D.R., & McGregor, K.C. (1999). Racial differences in the multiple social roles of older women: Implications for depressive symptoms. *The Gerontologist, 39*, 465-472.

Cooper, L.A., Brown, C., Vu, H. T., Ford, D., & Powe, N. (2001). How important is intrinsic spirituality in depression care? *Journal of General Internal Medicine, 16*, 634.

Crowther, M., Parker, M.W., Koenig, H., Larimore, W., & Achenbaum, A. (2002). Rowe and Kahn's model of successful aging revisited: Spirituality the forgotten factor. *The Gerontologist, 42*, 613-620.

Eaton, W., & Kessler, R. (1981). Rates of symptoms of depression in a national sample. *American Journal of Epidemiology, 114*, 528-538.

Fiscella, K., & Franks, P. (1997). Does psychological distress contribute to racial and socioeconomic disparities in mortality? *Social Science & Medicine, 45*, 1805-1809.

Gallo, J.J., Cooper-Patrick, L., & Lesikar, S. (1998). Depressive symptoms of whites and African Americans aged 60 years and older. *Journals of Gerontology Series B: Psychological Sciences and Social Sciences, 53*, P277-P286.

Gallo, J.J., & Lebowitz, B.D. (1999). The epidemiology of common late-life mental disorders in the community: Themes for the new century. *Psychiatric Services, 50*, 1158-1166.

George, L.K. (2002). The links between religion and health: Are they real? *Public Policy and Aging Report, 12*, 1, 3-6.

Gurland, B.J., Cross, P.S., & Katz, S. (1996). Epidemiological perspectives on opportunities for treatment of depression. *American Journal of Geriatric Psychiatry, 4*(Suppl. 1), S7-S13.

Hays, J.C., Landerman, L.R., George, L.K., Flint, E.P., Koenig, H.G., Land, K.C. et al. (1998). Social correlates of the dimensions of depression in the elderly. *Journals of Gerontology Series B: Psychological Sciences and Social Sciences, 53*, P31-39.

Hybels, C.F., Blazer, D.G., & Pieper, C.F. (2001). Toward a threshold for subthreshold depression: An analysis of correlates of depression by severity of symptoms using data from an elderly community sample. *The Gerontologist, 41*, 357-365.

Idler, E.L. (1987). Religious involvement and the health of the elderly: Some hypotheses and an initial test. *Social Forces, 66*, 226-238.

Idler, E.L. (2002). The many causal pathways linking religion to health. *Public Policy and Aging Report, 12*, 7-12.

Idler, E.L., Kasl, S., & Hays, J. (2001). Patterns of religious practice and belief in the last year of life. *Journals of Gerontology Series B: Psychological and Social Sciences, 56B*, S326-334.

Kendler, K.S., Gardner, C.O., & Prescott, C.A. (1997). Religion, psychopathology, and substance use and abuse. A multimeasure, genetic-epidemiologic study. *American Journal of Psychiatry, 154*, 322-329.

Kennedy, G., Kelman, H., Thomas, C., Wisniewsky, W., Metz, H., & Bijur, P. (1989). Hierarchy of characteristics associated with depressive symptoms in an urban elderly sample. *American Journal of Psychiatry, 146*, 220-225.

Kockler, M., & Huen, R. (2002). Gender differences of depressive symptoms in depressed and nondepressed elderly persons. *International Journal of Geriatric Psychiatry, 17*, 65-72.

Koenig, H.G., Cohen, H.J., Blazer, D.G., Kudler, H.S., Krishnan, K.R.R., & Sibert, T.E. (1995). Religious coping and cognitive symptoms of depression in elderly medical patients. *Psychosomatics, 36*, 369-375.

Koenig, H.G., Cohen, H.J., Blazer, D.G., Pieper, C., Meador, K.G., Shelp, F. et al. (1992). Religious coping and depression in elderly hospitalized medically ill men. *American Journal of Psychiatry, 149*, 1693-1700.

Koenig, H.G., & Futterman, A. (1995). Religion and health outcomes: A review and synthesis of the literature. In Proceedings of the Conference on Methodological Approaches to the Study of Religion, Aging, and Health, National Institute on Aging and the Fetzer Institute (March 16-17).

Koenig, H.G., Hays, J.C., George, L.K., Blazer, D.G., Larson, D.B., & Landerman, L.R. (1997a). Modeling the cross-sectional relationships between religion, physical health, social support, and depressive symptoms. *The American Journal of Geriatric Psychiatry*, 5, 131-144.

Koenig, H.G., McCullough, M.E., & Larson, D.B. (2001). *Handbook of religion and health*. Oxford: Oxford University Press.

Koenig H. G., Meador K., & Parkerson, G. (1997b). Religion index for psychiatric research: A 5-item measure for use in health outcome studies. *American Journal of Psychiatry*, 154, 885-886.

Larson, D.B., Sherrill, K.A., Lyons, J.S., Craigie, F.C., Thielman, S.B., Greenwold, M.A. et al. (1992). Associations between dimensions of religious commitment and mental health reported in the *American Journal of Psychiatry* and *Archives of General Psychiatry*: 1978-1989. *American Journal of Psychiatry*, 149, 557-559.

Lebowitz, B.D., Pearson, J.L., Schneider, L.S., Reynolds, C.F., Alexopoulos, G.S., Bruce, M.L. et al. (1997). Diagnosis and treatment of depression in late life: Consensus statement update. *The Journal of the American Medical Association*, 278, 1186-1190.

Martin, E.P., & Martin, J.M. (2002). *Spirituality and the black helping tradition in social work*. Washington, DC: NASW Press.

Mays, V.M. (1985). The black American and psychotherapy: The dilemma. *Psychotherapy: Theory, research, practice and training*, 22, 69-78.

Mays, V.M., Caldwell, C.H., & Jackson, J.S. (1996). Mental health symptoms and service utilization patterns of help-seeking among African American women. In H.W. Neighbors, & J.S. Jackson (Eds.), *Mental health in black America* (pp. 161-176). Thousand Oaks, CA: Sage.

Mitchell, J., Mathews, H.F., & Yesavage, J.A. (1993). A multidimensional examination of depression among the elderly. *Research on Aging*, 15, 198-219.

Mulsant, B.H., & Ganguli, M. (1999). Epidemiology and diagnosis of depression in late life. *Journal of Clinical Psychiatry*, 60, 9-15.

Musick, M.A., Blazer, D.G., & Hays, J.C. (2000). Religious activity, alcohol use, and depression in a sample of elderly Baptists. *Research on Aging*, 22, 91-116.

Musick, M.A., Koenig, H.G., Hays, J.C., & Cohen, H.J. (1998). Religious activity and depression among community-dwelling elderly persons with cancer: The moderating effect of race. *The Journals of Gerontology Series B: Psychological Sciences and Social Sciences*, 53, S218-S227.

Okwumabua, J.O., Baker, F.M., Wong, S.P., & Pilgram, B.O. (1997). Characteristics of depressive symptoms in elderly urban and rural African Americans. *Journals of Gerontology Series A: Biological Sciences and Medical Sciences*, 52, M241-M246.

O'Neill, G. (2002). *The state of aging and health in America*. Washington, DC: Gerontological Society of America and Merck Institute of Aging and Health.

Ploch, D.R., & Hastings, D.R. (1994). Graphic presentations of church attendance using general social survey data. *Journal for the Scientific Study of Religion*, 33, 16-33.

Ren, X.S., Kazis, L., & Meenan, R.F. (1999). Short-form Arthritis Impact Measurement Scales: Tests of reliability and validity among patients with osteoarthritis. *Arthritis Care Research*, 40: 1267-74.

Roberts, R.E., Kaplan, G.A., Shema, S.J., & Strawbridge, W.J. (1997). Prevalence and correlates of depression in an aging cohort: The Alameda County Study. *Journals of Gerontology Series B: Psychological Sciences and Social Sciences*, 52, S252-S258.

Smallegan, M. (1989). Level of depressive symptoms and life stresses for culturally diverse older adults. *The Gerontologist, 29,* 45-50.

Solari-Twadell, A., & McDermott, M.A. (1999). *Parish nursing: Promoting the whole person within faith communities.* Thousand Oaks, CA: Sage.

U.S. Bureau of the Census (2000). Projections of the total resident population by 5-year age groups, race and Hispanic origin with special age categories: Middle series 1999-2000; middle series 2050-2070.

Ware, J.E., Kosinski, M., & Keller, S.D. (1995). SF-12: How to score the SF-12 physical and mental health summary scales (2nd edition). Boston: The Health Institute, New England Medical Center.

Ware, J.E., Kosinski, M., & Keller, S.D. (1996). A 12-item short-form health survey: Construction of scales and preliminary tests of reliability and validity. *Medical Care, 34,* 220-233.

Yesavage, J. (2002). Geriatric depression scale. Retrieved January 12, 2003 from *http://www.stanford.edu/~yesavage/GDS.english.short.score.html.*

Religiousness/Spirituality and Subjective Well-Being Among Rural Elderly Whites, African Americans, and Native Americans

Dong Pil Yoon
Eun-Kyoung Othelia Lee

SUMMARY. Little attention has been paid to subjective well-being among non-White elderly in rural areas where medical resources and financial support are deficient. The present study assessed a rural community sample of 215 elderly comprising 85 Caucasians, 75 African Americans, and 55 Native Americans, to examine roles of spirituality/ religiousness on their subjective well-being. This study found ethnic differences in the reliance on religiosity/spirituality and a significant association between dimensions of religiousness/spirituality and subjective well-being among all ethnic rural elderly groups. The results

Dong Pil Yoon, PhD, is Assistant Professor, University of Missouri-Columbia, School of Social Work, 701 Clark Hall, Columbia, MO 65211 (E-mail: yoond@missouri.edu). Eun-Kyoung Othelia Lee, PhD, is Assistant Professor, Boston College, Graduate School of Social Work, McGuinn Hall #206, Chestnut Hill, MA 02467 (E-mail: othelia.lee@ bc.edu).

We would like to express our thanks to Dr. Judith Davenport for her continuous assistance and insightful comments on our research.

[Haworth co-indexing entry note]: "Religiousness/Spirituality and Subjective Well-Being Among Rural Elderly Whites, African Americans, and Native Americans." Yoon, Dong Pil, and Eun-Kyoung Othelia Lee. Co-published simultaneously in *Journal of Human Behavior in the Social Environment* (The Haworth Social Work Practice Press, an imprint of The Haworth Press, Inc.) Vol. 10, No. 1, 2004, pp. 191-211; and: *Diversity and Aging in the Social Environment* (eds: Sherry M. Cummings, and Colleen Galambos) The Haworth Social Work Practice Press, an imprint of The Haworth Press, Inc., 2004, pp. 191-211. Single or multiple copies of this article are available for a fee from The Haworth Document Delivery Service [1-800-HAWORTH, 9:00 a.m. - 5:00 p.m. (EST). E-mail address: docdelivery@haworthpress.com].

of the study suggest that health providers, social workers, and faith communities need to provide rural elderly with religious and spiritual support in order to enhance their life satisfaction and lessen their emotional distress. *[Article copies available for a fee from The Haworth Document Delivery Service: 1-800-HAWORTH. E-mail address: <docdelivery@haworthpress.com> Website: <http://www.HaworthPress.com> © 2004 by The Haworth Press, Inc. All rights reserved.]*

KEYWORDS. Religiousness/spirituality, subjective well-being, rural elderly, Native American elderly, African American elderly

INTRODUCTION

A growing number of interdisciplinary studies explores the role of religiosity and spirituality on quality of life, mental health and general well-being among older adults. In particular, gerontologists and geriatricians have focused on the health and mental health effects of religiousness/spirituality, acknowledging that religiousness/spirituality is a profoundly important personal resource for older adults in terms of an intrapsychic means of coping and adaptation with issues of daily life, change, loss, and death. Empirical studies strongly support that there is a positive effect of religion on health and general well-being among older adults (Commerford & Reznikoff, 1996; Idler & Kasl, 1997; Koenig et al., 1997; Oman & Reed, 1998; Koenig & Larson, 1998). There is also mounting evidence linking spirituality with positive well-being among older adults (Levin & Chatters, 1998; Fry, 2000; Fabricatore, Handal, & Fenzel, 2000). Although a large body of literature suggests that religiousness/spirituality has beneficial implications for physical and mental health, few studies focus on minority elderly in rural areas where medical resources and health care are limited and emergency financial assistance and community support are deficient. In this study, the researchers compare and contrast degrees of religious and spiritual aspects among three ethnic elderly groups (White, African American, and Native American) in rural areas as well as examine the relationship between religiousness/spirituality and subjective well-being among them.

LITERATURE REVIEW

Characteristics of Life Among Minority Elderly

The older population in the United States is predominantly White, but as the older population increases, it is becoming more racially and ethnically diverse. Minority populations are projected to represent 25.5% of the elderly population in 2030, up from 16.1% in 1999. Between 1999 and 2030, the White population 65+ is projected to increase by 81% compared with 219% for older minorities (U.S. Census Bureau, 1999). Despite their growing numbers, in terms of socioeconomic status, the majority of minority elderly have more disadvantages than White elderly. For instance, approximately 33% of African American elderly live in poverty, and nearly one-half of them live at or below the poverty level in rural areas. More than half of African American elderly are in poor health and experience higher rates of multiple chronic illnesses than the rest of the population (Jackson, 1988). Relative to the general population, Native American elderly are economically disadvantaged (AARP, 1987), and the overall life expectancy of the Native American is shorter than that of all other races (National Indian Council on Aging, 1981). Researchers have come to the conclusion that Native American elderly are at risk for an array of mental health problems including depression (Manson, 1995; Lichtenberg et al., 1997; McFall et al., 2000; Baldridge, 2001). An increasing number of studies observed racial disparities in the use of social resources and health services among older adults (Lee et al., 1998; Auchincloss, van Nostrand, & Ronsaville, 2001; Dunlop et al., 2002). Research has consistently documented that minority elderly have poorer health than do Whites due to poverty, a lack of access to and utilization of health care, and the encountering of inadequate cultural competence by health providers and programs (AARP, 1987).

Characteristics of Life Among Rural Elderly

In general, rural areas have a higher proportion of older adults in their total population (20%) than do urban areas (15%) (Rogers, 2002). Rural communities are often characterized as small-scale, with low density population, and a paucity of transportation, social services, and medical facilities (Kaufman et al., 2000). Due to these factors and traditional cultural belief systems, older adults residing in rural areas are at a greater disadvantage (Arcury et al., 2000; Bane & Bull, 2001). Rural older adults generally have less education, higher poverty rates, poorer health, and higher mortality rates than urban older adults (Buczko, 2001; Rogers, 2002). Dellasega (1998) found that although rural older adults were not necessarily in poorer self-reported health, these elderly were significantly poorer in objective health as measured by the number of reported symptoms. Despite having a greater number of specific health complaints, these rural individuals did not use significantly more services or report more unmet needs. Rural residents rely heavily on social networks to provide social support and other services that more formal agencies often provide in urban areas (Davenport & Davenport, 1982). Many rural residents are highly religious and are more likely to turn to their pastors and religious leaders for help with emotional, mental, and relational problems (Campbell, Gordon, & Chandler, 2002).

Roles of Religiousness/Spirituality Among Diverse Elderly

Researchers identified religious and spiritual effects on many psychosocial and health-related outcomes in older adults. Mostly positive effects were found in relation to subjective well-being (Levin & Markides, 1986; Poloma & Pendleton, 1990), dimensions of psychological well-being such as life satisfaction (Anson, Antonovsky, & Sagy, 1990; Levin, Chatters, & Taylor, 1995), and depressive symptoms (McClure & Loden, 1982; Hertsgaard & Light, 1984; Koenig, Moberg, & Kvale, 1988; Koenig et al., 1997). These findings suggest that religious involvement may benefit the lives of older adults through enhancing internal psychological resources such as feelings of self-esteem and worthiness and by providing concrete social resources such as religious fellowship and congregational networks (Ellison, 1994). However, as the association between religiousness/spirituality and mental health may be affected by the larger social context, the effects of religiousness/spirituality on subjective well-being among older adults may vary systematically by factors such as race and region.

African American elderly. Religious practices, rituals, and beliefs may provide specific coping resources for African Americans. The research by Neighbors et al. (1983) confirms that a large percentage of African Americans turn to prayer in coping with serious personal problems, and express considerable satisfaction with the results of religious coping strategies. Black et al. (1998) and Black (1999) found that rural poor African American elderly relied on religious consolation, and attributed their ability to cope with difficulties to a strong faith in God's ability to sustain them. Research supports that there is a positive relationship between religious involvement and life satisfaction among elder African Americans (Heisel & Faulkner, 1982; Levin & Vanderpool, 1989; Coke, 1992; Bryant & Rakowski, 1992; Ellison, 1994; Levin, Chatters, & Taylor, 1995). Using a national sample of African Americans, Ellison and Gay (1990) documented that religious participation was positively associated with subjective well-being only among non-southern African Americans. Krause and Tran (1989) also found that aspects of religious involvement were positively associated with self-esteem, personal mastery, and the sense of control over one's affairs among African Americans.

Several studies suggest that religiousness/spirituality may play a different role according to race. Mitchell and Weatherly (2000) indicate that Christian religious beliefs and practices are widespread in mainly rural populations and that African American older adults are more likely than White older adults to profess religious beliefs and to participate in church-based activities. Musick et al. (1998) found that the effects of religious activity were stronger among Blacks than Whites. A study by Koenig (1998) reported that religious variables were consistently and independently related to being Black, having lower education, and greater life stressors. Religious variables were also related to stronger social support systems, and religious attendance was associated with less medical illness. Several analyses of data indicate that religious involvement generally bears a stronger positive relationship with life satisfaction and other aspects of subjective well-being for African Americans than for Whites of similar backgrounds (St. George & McNamara, 1984; Thomas & Holmes, 1992).

Native American elderly. By and large, religion and spirituality may give rise to Native American values and shape how Native Americans function in daily life (Toelken, 1976). According to Bryde (1971), the majority of Native American values and actions relate to universal realities that historically were important to the culture. For example, the spiritual God of the Native Americans is positive, benevolent, and part of daily living (Axelson, 1985). Health and wholeness, whether physical, social, mental, or spiritual, depends on keeping harmonious relationships with the spirit world (Matheson, 1996). The Native American Church (NAC) is considered by some to represent a blending of Christianity and traditional Native practices. Some Native Americans have not adopted Christianity at all and continue to practice their own forms of religion and spirituality. Some combine aspects of both indigenous spirituality and Christianity; whereas others abandon their spiritual traditions and are fully assimilated into western culture, including Christianity. Despite the image that Native Americans have a strong spiritual belief system, little attention has been paid to studying the role of spirituality/religiousness on the health and well-being among Native American elderly.

Building on this literature review, the purpose of this study is to compare and contrast degrees of religious and spiritual aspects among three ethnic elderly groups, including White, African American, and Native American, in rural areas as well as to examine the relationship between religiousness/spirituality and subjective well-being among them.

METHODS

Sample and Data Collection

A convenience sample of 215 older adults was obtained at local senior centers in eight counties in both West Virginia and North Carolina in 2002. To ensure adequate representation of the diverse racial/ethnic groups, the quota sampling method was used, resulting in 85 Caucasians, 75 African Americans, and 55 Native Americans dwelling in rural communities. Each participant was interviewed through structured questionnaires at local senior centers. These interviews were 40-50 minutes in duration and were conducted by the research assistants who had working experience with older adults. Each participant had an ability to understand and answer the questions. At the beginning of each interview, the interviewer explained the purpose and format of the interview, emphasizing the confidentiality of all information collected. All participants signed a detailed informed consent form, and all responses were completely voluntary and anonymous.

Measures

Religiousness/Spirituality. To measure various domains of religiousness/spirituality, as a short form, the Brief Multidimensional Measures of Religiousness/Spirituality (Fetzer/NIA, 1999) was used. For this study, researchers selected six subscales including daily spiritual experiences, values/beliefs, forgiveness, private religious practice, religious/spiritual coping, and religious support.

Daily spiritual experience measures the individual's perception of the transcendent (God, the divine) in daily life and perception of interaction with God. This subscale consisted of six items and a 5-point response format was used, which ranged from 1 (never) to 5 (everyday). Cronbach's alpha was .91 in the current sample.

*Values/beliefs*measures religious value and belief systems. A study reveals that many patients shape their personal responses to illness on the basis of their religious and spiritual beliefs; such beliefs play a major role in the decisions that they make about specific treatments (Larimore, 2001). This subscale consisted of two items and a 4-point response format was used, which ranged from 1 (strongly disagree) to 4 (strongly agree). Cronbach's alpha was .64 in the present sample.

Forgiveness measures the degree of forgiveness of self, others, and by God. This subscale consisted of three items rated on a 4-point response format, ranging from 1 (never) to 4 (always). Cronbach's alpha was .64 for this sample.

Private religious practice measures behaviors constituting the larger construct of religious involvement. This subscale consisted of five items rated on a 5-point response format, ranging from 1 (never) to 5 (everyday). Cronbach's alpha was .72 in the present sample.

Religious/spiritual coping (skill) measures religious/spiritual methods for coping with life's problems. Religious coping behaviors, including prayer, inspirational reading, participating in worship services, and seeking support from clergy or congregational members have been associated with the health and mental health related outcomes of a wide variety of critical life situations (Pargament et al., 1998). This subscale consisted of seven items and a 5-point response format was used, which ranged from 1 (not at all) to 5 (a great deal). Cronbach's alpha was .81 for this sample.

Religious support measures aspects of the social relationships between respondents and others in their shared place of worship. This subscale consisted of four items and a 4-point response format was used, which ranged from 1 (none) to 5 (very often). Cronbach's alpha was .72 in the current sample.

Subjective well-being. For this study subjective well-being was conceptualized as consisting of two dimensions: depression and life satisfaction. The Center for Epidemiological Studies-Depression (CES-D) (Radloff, 1977) and the Satisfaction with Life Scale (SWLS) (Diener et al., 1985) were used to measure subjective well-being. Cronbach's alphas for these two scales were .85 and .84, respectively, for this sample. The CES-D has been used to assess depressive symptomatology in the general population. The SWLS measures the degree of positive psychological well-being. The CES-D consisted of 11 items rated on a 4-point response format, ranging from 1 (rare or none of the time: less than a day) to 4 (most of the time: 5-7 days); and the SWLS consisted of five items rated on a 4-point response format, ranging from 1 (strongly disagree) to 4 (strongly agree).

Data Analyses

A one-way analysis of variance (ANOVA) was used to explore ethnic group differences in scores of religiousness and spirituality. For each ethnic elderly group (White, African American, and Native American), multiple regression analyses were performed to determine the relative influence of religiousness/spirituality on the dependent variable: subjective well-being including life satisfaction and depression. In particular, in order to consider a variety of religious and spiritual aspects, all six variables including daily spiritual experience, values and beliefs, forgiveness, private religious practice, spiritual coping, and religious support were used to determine the level of subjective well-being consisting of life satisfaction and depression. In addition, demographic variables were included as independent variables. In these analyses, the demographic variables consisted of age, gender (dichotomously coded as 1 = male, 0 = female), education (dichotomously coded as 1 = ≥ HS diploma, 0 = ≤ HS diploma), annual income (dichotomously coded as 1 = ≥ $10,000, 0 = ≤ $10,000), and living arrangement (dichotomously coded as 1 = living with someone, 0 = living alone).

RESULTS

Demographic Differences Among Three Ethnic Elderly Groups

Overall, females and males comprised approximately 62% and 38%, of the participants, respectively. The mean age of the respondents was 72-years-old with a range from 60 to 92 years. Most participants (97%) were affiliated with some type of religion: 185 being Protestant (88%), eight being Catholic (4%), and ten (5%) being affiliated with other religions and/or denominations. Annual income categories included 68 individuals reporting under $10,001 (31%), 78 reporting between $10,001-$20,000 (51%), and 69 individuals reporting over $20,000 (18%), indicating that about the majority of the participants are financially below or near the poverty line (DHHS, 2003).

Demographic characteristics are shown in Table 1 for older adults in three ethnic groups. There were statistically significant differences between the three groups in marital status, education, annual income, and living arrangement. In terms of education, about 67% of Native American elderly and almost 53% of African American elderly had no high school diploma, indicating that the majority of Non-White elderly had

TABLE 1. Comparison of Demographic Characteristics by Ethnic Group

Variable	White (n = 85)	African American (n = 75)	Native American (n = 55)	Test Statistics (χ^2)
Marital status (%)				25.97*
Married	42.4	32.4	18.2	
Widowed	28.2	39.2	63.6	
Divorced	12.9	6.8	3.6	
Single	12.9	16.2	14.5	
Other	3.6	5.4	0.1	
Education (%)				47.75***
Some high school	18.1	53.3	67.3	
High school diploma	31.3	32.0	16.4	
Some college	31.3	10.7	7.3	
College graduate	14.5	2.7	5.5	
Above college graduate	4.8	1.3	3.5	
Annual income (%)				26.48***
Under $10,001	14.1	38.0	32.7	
$10,001 to $20,000	53.8	52.7	52.7	
$20,001 to $30,000	25.0	8.3	9.1	
Over $30,000	7.1	1.0	5.5	
Religion (%)				15.99
Protestant	85.5	89.5	83.5	
Catholic	8.4	1.4	0.0	
Other	2.4	7.0	14.7	
No	3.7	2.1	1.8	
Living arrangement (%)				14.84**
Living alone	46.4	41.1	74.5	
Living with someone	53.6	58.9	25.5	

*p < .05; **p < .01; ***p < .001.

lower education; whereas about 82% of White elderly had at least a high school diploma. With respect to annual income, the majority of both African American elderly (90.7%) and Native American elderly (85.4%) reported less than $20,000 income, reflecting that the majority of Non-White elderly were financially poor; whereas about 32% of White elderly reported income greater than $20,000. Compared with other ethnic groups, the majority of Native American elderly lived alone (74.5%). Regardless of their ethnic backgrounds, most participants were religious with Protestant being the primary religious affiliation.

Ethnic Differences Among Religiousness/Spirituality and Subjective Well-Being

Six variables involving daily spiritual experience, values/beliefs, forgiveness, private religious practice, religious/spiritual coping, and religious support were used to measure religiousness/spirituality (see Table 2). Daily spiritual experience scores ranged from 6 (never) to 30 (everyday) with a mean of 24.6, showing that respondents reported experiencing spiritually most days. There were no ethnic group differences in spiritual experiences. Respondents agreed to having strong religious value and belief in a God (Mean = 6.5), ranging from 2 (strongly disagree) to 8 (strongly agree). There were no ethnic group differences in values and beliefs.

Forgiveness scores ranged from 4 (never) to 12 (always) with a mean of 10.1, indicating that often respondents reported experiencing forgiveness. There were significant ethnic group differences in forgiveness, $F(2, 16) = 8.21$, $p < .001$. The Scheffe test revealed that African American elderly had higher scores on forgiveness than did White elderly.

Respondents reported practicing religious activities a couple of days during a week (Mean = 19.2), ranging from 5 (never) to 25 (daily). There were significant ethnic group differences in religious practice, $F(2, 398) = 19.73$, $p < .001$, with the Scheffe test revealing that both African American and Native American elderly practiced more religious activities than did White elderly.

Religious and spiritual coping scores ranged from 7 (not at all) to 28 (a great deal) with a mean of 19.2, indicating that respondents reported using considerable religious and spiritual coping skills. There were also ethnic differences in religious and spiritual coping, $F(2, 442) = 42.02$, $p < .001$. The Scheffe test revealed that Native American elderly used more religious and spiritual coping skills than did both African American and White elderly. Simultaneously, African American elderly used more religious and spiritual coping skills than did White elderly.

Respondents reported receiving some religious support (Mean = 10.5), ranging from 4 (none) to 16 (a great deal). There were significant ethnic group differences in religious support, $F(2, 84) = 20.30$, $p < .001$, with the Scheffe test revealing that Native American elderly received more religious support than did both African American and White elderly.

The two variables of depression and life satisfaction were used to measure subjective well-being. Depression scores ranged from 11

TABLE 2. One-Way Analysis of Variance of Ethnic Group Differences in Religiousness/Spirituality and Subjective Well-Being

Variable	White (n = 85)		African American (n = 75)		Native American (n = 55)		Total (n = 215)		F test
	M	SD	M	SD	M	SD	M	SD	
Religiousness/spirituality									
Spiritual experiences	24.28	4.87	25.13	4.23	24.19	2.51	24.56	4.15	1.10
Values and beliefs	6.59	1.31	6.33	1.18	6.55	0.77	6.49	1.15	1.13
Forgiveness	9.67	1.31	10.57	1.54	10.04	1.37	10.08	1.46	8.22***
Private religious practice	17.72	5.57	21.65	4.10	21.68	2.85	20.10	4.87	19.73***
Religious and spiritual coping	17.13	2.86	19.31	3.65	22.27	3.20	19.20	3.82	42.02***
Religious support	10.53	1.72	9.96	2.72	12.04	1.20	10.53	2.21	20.30***
Subjective well-being									
Depression	19.84	4.68	20.88	4.94	20.26	2.25	20.31	4.30	1.18
Life satisfaction	14.54	2.57	14.03	3.30	15.33	2.40	14.56	2.67	3.87*

*p < .05; **p < .01; ***p < .001.

(rarely) to 44 (most of the times) with a mean of 20.3, and life satisfaction scores ranged from 5 (strongly disagree) to 20 (strongly agree) with a mean of 14.6, showing that respondents exhibited slightly higher depressive symptoms and moderate levels of life satisfaction. There were no ethnic differences in depression. However, the Scheffe test revealed that Native American elderly had higher levels of life satisfaction than did African American elderly, $F(2, 27) = 3.87$, $p < .05$, indicating that there were ethnic group differences in life satisfaction.

Multivariate Analyses

Life satisfaction. As evidenced in Table 3, the regression model for White elderly accounted for 19% of the variance in life satisfaction. Among the demographic information, age was the only factor to significantly predict life satisfaction, reflecting that the older the respondents, the greater the life satisfaction. In the equation to predict life satisfaction, religiosity and spirituality did not appear to contribute significantly among White elderly individuals. For African American elderly, religious/spiritual coping skills and religious beliefs/values were significantly predictive of life satisfaction, explaining 31% of the variance in life satisfaction. It seems likely that African American elderly reporting higher levels of life satisfaction could possess more religious/spiritual coping skills and strong religious beliefs/values. The regression model for Native American elderly accounted for 30% of the variance in life satisfaction. Forgiveness significantly predicted life satisfaction, indicating that Native American elderly who were high in life satisfaction were more likely to experience forgiveness. Consequently, religiosity and spirituality were statistically significant as positive predictors of life satisfaction among non-White elderly, specifically African American and Native American elderly.

Depression. As can be seen in Table 3, the results of the regression analysis on depression have been summarized. Indicators of socioeconomic status failed to significantly predict depression among all ethnic groups. For White elderly, religious/spiritual coping skills, religious beliefs/values, and forgiveness were significant predictors of depression, explaining 29% of the variance in depression. Thus, those White elderly reporting lower levels of depression were more likely to have more religious/spiritual coping skills, possess strong religious values/beliefs, and experience forgiveness. The regression model for African American elderly accounted for 20% of the variance of depression. Forgiveness was a significant predictor of depression, reflecting that African American elderly experiencing more forgiveness were likely to indicate lower levels of depression. In the equa-

TABLE 3. Summary of Regression Analyses for Variables Predicting Subjective Well-Being Among Three Ethnic Groups (Standardized Beta Coefficients)

Variable	White (n = 85)		African American (n = 75)		Native American (n = 55)	
	Life Satisfaction	Depression	Life Satisfaction	Depression	Life Satisfaction	Depression
Demographic Information						
Age	.22*	.00	.09	-.03	.17	-.13
Gender	-.01	-.02	.07	-.07	.20	-.20
Education	.04	-.15	.03	.00	.09	-.01
Annual income	.08	-.02	.21	-.05	.06	-.15
Living arrangement	.10	-.17	.11	.00	.10	-.12
Religiousness/spirituality						
Spiritual experiences	.06	.04	.12	.05	.25	-.17
Values and beliefs	.15	-.38*	.24*	-.09	.10	.01
Forgiveness	.01	-.28*	.13	-.39*	.33*	-.07
Private religious practice	-.06	.06	.18	.07	.11	-.15
Religious and spiritual coping	.20	-.23*	.40*	-.17	.12	-.41**
Religious support	.14	.00	.10	-.09	-.10	.05
R^2	.19	.29	.31	.20	.30	.39

* p < .05, ** p < .01, *** p < .001.

203

tion to predict depression among Native American elderly, religious and spiritual coping skills appeared to contribute significantly, explaining 39% of the variance in depression. Native American elderly who were less depressed were more likely to use religious and spiritual coping skills. Therefore, religiosity and spirituality were statistically significant as negative predictors of depression among all ethnic groups.

DISCUSSION

Regardless of ethnic background, the results of this study demonstrate the importance of several dimensions of religiousness/spirituality in the prediction of subjective well-being in rural community-residing older adults. In accordance with findings of previous studies on older adults in urban/metropolitan areas (Anson, Antonovsky, & Sagy, 1990; Coke, 1992; Bryant & Rakowski, 1992; Levin, Chatters, & Taylor, 1995), multiple regression analyses found that religiosity and spirituality were significantly related to subjective well-being among rural elderly individuals. However, these analyses found that there was no significant impact of demographic information on subjective well-being.

Consistent with previous studies (Ellison & Gay, 1990; Levin, Chatters, & Taylor, 1995), the multiple regression analyses with this study indicate that religiosity and spirituality are important for life satisfaction of African American elderly. More specifically, the combined impact of religious/spiritual coping skills and religious beliefs/values produced a greater life satisfaction. Like other studies (Neighbors et al., 1983; Black, 1999), spirituality/religiousness played a significant role in decreasing levels of depression. It was apparent that religiosity and spirituality were resources that enhanced levels of life satisfaction and lowered levels of depression among rural Native American elderly. This finding was similar to previous findings related to African American elderly. The lack of a significant relationship between spirituality/religiousness and life satisfaction among White elderly was surprising in view of previous studies showing a significant relationship between religiosity and life satisfaction among White elderly individuals. However, spirituality/religiousness played a significant role in decreasing levels of depression among White elderly. Therefore, this study confirmed previous findings that the effects of spirituality and religiosity were stronger among non-White elderly than White elderly. The overall findings of multiple regression analyses support a growing body of literature documenting the importance of religiousness/spirituality as a supportive resource for affirming psychological well-being in late life.

The results of ANOVA also revealed that significant differences were found in levels of religiousness/spirituality between White and non-White elderly. Specifically, Native American elderly experienced more spiritual and religious activities than did both African American and White elderly. In accordance with prior research (St. George & McNamara, 1984; Thomas & Holmes, 1992), African American elderly engaged in more religious/spiritual practices than did White elderly. These findings demonstrate that non-White elderly are more likely to be religious and spiritual than their White peers, which suggests that an attachment to religious and spiritual activities is very prominent among non-White elderly in rural areas.

This research differs from previous studies in that it examines variables predicting subjective well-being in rural areas. Most of the previous studies investigating the relationship between health/mental health and religiousness/spirituality have been conducted among elderly in urban or metropolitan areas where medical resources, health care services, and community support are more accessible and more sufficient than in rural areas. Another difference is that previous studies used a unidimensional construct. This study was unique in that it attempted to capture the multidimensional aspects of religiousness/spirituality as a significant role in the enhancement of subjective well-being among rural elderly, detecting the ethnic differences along specific dimensions of religiosity and spirituality through the use of the multidimensional construct. It is hypothesized that, by gaining insight into how each dimension (daily spiritual experience, values and beliefs, forgiveness, private religious practice, spiritual coping, and religious support) uniquely works, the importance of each dimension is verified more thoroughly. Thus, a clearer picture is obtained among the differences between these groups due to the use of multidimensional aspects of religiousness/spirituality. It is notable that this is the first exploratory study of religious and spiritual effects on subjective well-being among Native American elderly.

Limitations and Suggestions for the Future Study

The limitations of the present study should be considered when interpreting these findings. The small nonprobability sample in this study limited the ability to generalize to the population as a whole. In addition, a potential selection bias may have been created by excluding elderly individuals with different socioeconomic backgrounds and value/belief systems from other geographic locations around the states. As the present study was limited by its cross-sectional design, it is recommended that a longitudinal design with a larger random sample be conducted to understand the functions of spirituality/religiousness on subjective well-being over different life-courses according to race. In particular, more research in the area of religious and spiritual effects on general well-being among Native American elderly is needed due to the current lack of available research in this area.

Implications for Social Work Practice

In spite of these limitations, findings of this study can provide significant implications for health providers and social workers. Given the evidence concerning significant influence of religion and spirituality on subjective well-being, practitioners should routinely include assessment of spirituality and religious practices when working with diverse groups of older adults. Having knowledge about the spiritual resources of the patient prior to the sudden worsening or onset of a medical condition is always preferable to having to initiate a spiritual assessment at the time of the acute event. If the elderly individual is relying on religious beliefs and spiritual practices to cope, intervention by a health care provider that acknowledges and strengthens those beliefs is more likely to bolster his/her ability to cope. Helping elderly patients to forgive can reduce their level of hurt, anger, and perceived offense and improve their mood and emotional status (Harris et al., 1999). Spirituality-informed interventions focusing on spiritual perspectives should be provided in order to be congruent with expectancies of life quality of the religiously-oriented elderly.

Health care providers need to be sensitive to elders' faith development so that a spiritual dimension can be integrated in assessment and intervention. Elderly clients are, therefore, encouraged to discuss their religious and spiritual life and to explore what it means to them to be involved in their faith communities. Simultaneously, faith communities need to work closely with mental health professionals in providing environments that support the spiritual growth of elderly individuals. Religious and spiritual communities can be the source of support for clients because they can provide a sense of belonging, safety, purpose, and opportunities for giving and receiving service (Richard & Bergin, 1997).

In particular, the results of this study can help service providers to understand and evaluate the impact of religion and spirituality in various ethnic groups of older adults in order to improve quality of life. For instance, the holistic view of mind, body, and spirit among Native American elderly is important in health intervention. Thus, culturally-sensitive intervention and outreach approaches should take into account the importance of faith and faith-based communities for ethnic minority elderly in the rural areas. Ethnic minority elderly should be encouraged to collaborate with their faith-based communities in order to design interventions that integrate spirituality into educational and clinical modalities.

In conclusion, successful rural models of mental health care need to be based on information that is germane to rural community life, such as specific training of mental health professionals to work in rural settings, the engagement of rural older adults as peer counselors in outreach, and the need for strong linkages with existing services and programs. Findings of this study suggest that social workers and other health care professionals develop programs or services aimed at promoting religious or spiritual growth and that assist in enhancing the quality of life and in improving general well-being of elderly individuals in rural areas.

REFERENCES

American Association of Retired Persons (AARP) (1987). *A portrait of older minorities.* Washington, DC: AARP.

Anson, O., Antonovsky, A., & Sagy, S. (1990). Religiosity and well-being among retirees: A question of causality, *Behavior, Health, & Aging, 1*(2), 85-97.

Arcury, T. A., Quandt, S. A., McDonald, J., & Bell, R. A. (2000). Faith and health self-management of rural older adults. *Journal of Cross-Cultural Gerontology, 15*(1), 55-74.

Auchincloss, A. H., van Nostrand, J. F., & Ronsaville, D. (2001). Access to health care for older persons in the United States. *Journal of Aging and Health, 13*(3), 329-354.

Axelson, J. A. (1985). *Counseling and development in a multicultural society.* Monterey, CA: Brooks/Cole Publishing.

Baker, D. C., & Nussbaum, P. D. (1997). Religious practice and spirituality then and now: A retrospective study of spiritual dimensions of residents residing at a continuing care retirement community. *Journal of Religious Gerontology, 10*(3), 33-51.

Baldridge, D. (2001). Elder Indian population and long-term care. In Dixon-Mim & Roubideaux-Yvette (Eds.), *Promises to keep: Public health policy for American Indians and Alaska Natives in the 21st century* (pp. 137-164). Washington, DC: American Public Health Association.

Bane, S. D., & Bull, C. N. (2001). Innovative rural mental health service delivery for rural elders. *Journal of Applied Gerontology, 20*(2), 230-240.

Black, B. S., Rabins, P. V., German, P., Roca, R., McGuire, M., & Brant, L. J. (1998). Use of formal and informal sources of mental health care among older African-American public-housing residents. *Psychological Medicine, 28,* 519-530.

Black, H. K. (1999). Poverty and prayer: Spiritual narratives of elderly African-American women. *Review of Religious Research, 40*(4), 359-374.

Bryant, S., & Rakowski, W. (1992). Predictors of mortality among elderly African-Americans. *Research on Aging, 14*(1), 50-67.

Bryde, J. F. (1971). *Indian students and guidance.* Oxford, England: Houghton Mifflin.

Buczko, W. (2001). Rural Medicare beneficiaries' use of rural and urban hospitals. *Journal of Rural Health, 17*(1), 53-58.

Campbell, C. D., Gordon, M. C., & Chandler, A. A. (2002). Wide open spaces: Meeting mental health needs in underserved rural areas. *Journal of Psychology & Christianity, 21*(4), 325-332.

Coke, M. M. (1992). Correlates of life satisfaction among elderly African Americans. *Journal of Gerontology, 47*(5), P316-P320.

Commerford, M. C., & Reznikoff, M. (1996). Relationship of religion and perceived social support to self-esteem and depression in nursing home residents. *Journal of Psychology, 130*(1), 35-50.

Davenport, J., & Davenport III, J. (1982). Utilizing the social network in rural communities. *Social Casework, 63,* 106-115.

Dellasega, C. (1998). Assessment of cognition in the elderly: Pieces of a complex puzzle. *Nursing Clinics of North America, 33*(3), 395-405.

DHHS (2003). The 2003 HHS poverty guidelines. *Federal Register, 68*(26), 6456-6458.

Diener, E., Emmons, R. A., Larsen, R. J., & Griffin, S. (1985). The satisfaction with life scale: A measure of life satisfaction. *Journal of Personality Assessment, 49,* 71-75.

Dunlop, D. D., Manheim, L. M., Song, J., & Chang, R. W. (2002). Gender and ethnic-racial disparities in health care utilization among older adults. *Journals of Gerontology: Series B: Psychological Sciences and Social Sciences, 57B*(4), S221-S233.

Ellison, C. G., & Gay, D. A. (1990). Region, religious commitment, and life satisfaction among Black Americans. *Sociological Quarterly, 31*(1), 123-147.

Ellison, C. G. (1994). Religion, the life stress paradigm, and the study of depression. In J. S. Levin (Ed.), *Religion in aging and health: Theoretical foundations and methodological frontiers* (pp. 78-121). Thousand Oaks, CA: Sage Publications.

Ellison, C. G. (1995). Rational choice explanations of individual religious behavior: Notes on the problem of social embeddedness. *Journal for the Scientific Study of Religion, 34*(1), 89-97.

Fabricatore, A. N., Handal, P. J., & Fenzel, L. M. (2000). Personal spirituality as a moderator of the relationship between stressors and subjective well-being. *Journal of Psychology & Theology, 28*(3), 221-228.

Fetzer Institute/National Institute on Aging (1999). *Multidimensional measurement of religiousness/spirituality for use in health research*: A report of the Fetzer Institute/National Institute on Aging working group. Kalamazoo, MI: John E. Fetzer Institute.

Fry, P. S. (2000). Religious involvement, spirituality and personal meaning for life: Existential predictors of psychological well-being in community-residing and institutional care elders. *Aging and Mental Health, 4*(4), 375-387.

Harris, A. H. S., Thoresen, C. E., McCullough, M. E., & Larson, D. B. (1999). Spiritually and religiously oriented health intervention. *Journal of Health Psychology, 4,* 413-433.

Heisel, M. A., & Faulkner, A. O. (1982). Religiosity in an older Black population. *The Gerontologist, 22,* 354-358.

Hertsgaard, D., & Light, H. K. (1984). Anxiety, depression, and hostility in rural women. *Psychological Reports, 55*(2), 673-674.

Idler, E. L., & Kasl, S. V. (1997). Religion among disabled and nondisabled persons I: Cross-sectional patterns in health practices, social activities, and well-being. *Journals of Gerontology: Series B: Psychological Sciences & Social Sciences, 52B*(6), S294-S305.

Idler, E. L., & Kast, S. V. (1997). Religion among disabled and nondisabled persons II: Attendance at religious services as a predictor of the course of disability. *Journals of Gerontology: Series B: Psychological Sciences & Social Sciences, 52B*(6), S306-S316.

Jackson, J. S. (1988). *The Black American elderly: Research on physical and psychosocial health.* New York: Springer.

Kaufman, A. V., Scogin, F. R., MaloneBeach, E. E., Baumhover, L. A., & McKendree-Smith, N. (2000). Home-delivered mental health services for aged rural home health care recipients. *Journal of Applied Gerontology, 19*(4), 460-475.

Koenig, H. G. (1998). Religious attitudes and practices of hospitalized medically ill older adults. *International Journal of Geriatric Psychiatry, 13*(4), 213-224.

Koenig, H. G., Cohen, H. J., George, L. K., Hays, J. C., Larson, D. B., & Blazer, D. G. (1997). Attendance at religious services, interleukin-6, and other biological indicators of immune function in older adults. *International Journal of Psychiatry in Medicine, 27,* 233-250.

Koenig, H. G., Hays, J. C., George, L. K., Blazer, D. G., Larson, D. B., & Landerman, L. R. (1997). Modeling the cross-sectional relationships between religion, physical health, social support, and depressive symptoms. *American Journal of Geriatric Psychiatry, 5,* 131-143.

Koenig, H. G., & Larson, D. B. (1998). Use of hospital services, religious attendance, and religious affiliation. *Southern Medical Journal, 91,* 925-932.

Koenig, H. G., Moberg, D. O., & Kvale, J. N. (1988). Religious activities and attitudes of older adults in a geriatric assessment clinic. *Journal of the American Geriatrics Society, 36*(4), 362-374.

Krause, N., & Tran, T. V. (1989). Stress and religious involvement among older Blacks. *Journal of Gerontology Social Science, 44,* S4-S13.

Larimore, W. L. (2001). Providing basic spiritual care for patients: Should it be the exclusive domain of pastoral professionals? *American Family Physician, 63*(1), 36-40.

Lee, A. J., Baker, C. S., Gehlbach, S., Hosmer, D. W., & Reti, M. (1998). Do black elderly Medicare patients receive fewer services? An analysis of procedure use for selected patient conditions. *Medical Care Research and Review, 55*(3), 314-333.

Levin, J. S., & Markides, K. S. (1986). Religious attendance and subjective health. *Journal of Scientific Study on Religion, 25,* 31-40.

Levin, J. S., & Vanderpool, H. Y. (1989). Religious factors in physical health and prevention of illness. In K. I. Pargament, K. I. Moton, & B. E. Hess (Ed.), *Religion and* prevention in mental health: Research, vision, and action (pp. 83-103). New York: The Haworth Press, Inc.

Levin, J. S., & Chatters, L. M. (1998). Religion, health, and psychological well-being in older adults. *Journal of Aging and Health, 10*(4), 504-531.

Levin, J. S., Chatters, L. M., & Taylor, R. J. (1995). Religious effect on health status. and life satisfaction among Black Americans. *Journal of Gerontology Social Sciences, 50B,* S134-S163.

Lichtenberg, P. A., Chapleski, E. E., & Youngblade, L. M. (1997). Effect of depression on functional abilities among Great Lakes American Indians. *Journal of Applied Gerontology, 16*(2), 235-248.

Manson, S. M. (1995). Mental health status and needs of the American Indian and Alaska native elderly. In D. K. Padgett (Ed.), *Handbook on ethnicity, aging, and mental health* (pp. 132-141). Westport, CT: Greenwood Press.

Matheson, L. (1996). Valuing spirituality among Native American populations. *Counseling & Values, 41*(1), 51-58.

McClure, R. F., & Loden, M. (1982). Religious activity, denomination membership and life satisfaction. *Journal of Human Behavior, 19*(1), 12-17.

McFall, S. L., Solomon, T. G. A., & Smith, D. W. (2000). Health-related quality of life of older Native American primary care patients. *Research on Aging, 22*(6), 692-714.

Mitchell, J., & Weatherly, D. (2000). Beyond church attendance: Religiosity and mental health among rural older adults. *Journal of Cross-Cultural Gerontology, 15*(1), 37-54.

Musick, M. A., Koenig, H. G., Hayes, J. C., & Cohen, H. J. (1998). Religious activity and depression among community-dwelling elderly persons with cancer: The moderating effect of race. *Journals of Gerontology: Series B: Psychological Sciences and Social Sciences, 53B*(4), S218-S227.

National Indian Council on Aging (NICOA) (1981). *American Indian elderly: A national profile by the National Indian Council on Aging.* Albuquerque, NM: NICOA.

Neighbors, H. W., Jackson, J. S., Bowman, P. J., & Gurin, G. (1983). Stress, coping, and Black mental health: Preliminary findings from a national study. *Prevention in Human Services, 2*(3), 5-29.

Oman, D., & Reed, D. (1998). Religion and mortality among the community-dwelling elderly. *American Journal of Public Health, 88*(10), 1469-1475.

Pargament, K. I., Smith, B. W., Koenig, H. G., & Perez, L. (1998). Patterns of positive and negative religious coping with major life stressors. *Journal for the Scientific Study of Religion, 37*(4), 710-724.

Poloma, M. M., & Pendleton, B. F. (1990). Religious domains and general well-being. *Social Indicators Research, 22*(3), 255-276.

Radloff, L. S. (1977). The Center for Epidemiological Studies Depression scale: A self-report depression scale for research in the general population. *Applied Psychological Measurement, 1,* 385-401.

Richard, P. S., & Bergin, A. E. (1997). Religious and spiritual assessment. In P. S. Richard & A. E. Bergin (Ed.), *A spiritual strategy for counseling and psychotherapy* (pp. 171-199). Washington DC: American Psychological Association.

Rogers, C. C. (2002). The older population in 21st century rural America. *Rural America, 17*(3), 25-35.

St. George, A., & McNamara, P. H. (1984). Religion, race and psychological well-being. *Journal for the Scientific Study of Religion, 23*(4), 351-363.

Thomas, M. E., & Holmes, B. J. (1992). Determinants of satisfaction for Blacks and Whites. *Sociological Quarterly, 33*(3), 459-472.

Toelken, B. (1976). How many sheep will it hold? In W. H. Capps (Ed.), *Seeing with a native eye* (p. 23). New York: Harper & Row.

U.S. Census Bureau (1999). Current population reports: Series P-25, No.1129: *Projections of the number of households and families in the United States: 1999 to 2030.* Washington DC: U. S. Government Printing Office.

Index

Numbers followed by "f" indicates figures; "t" following a page number indicates tabular material.

BOOK ORDER FORM!

Order a copy of this book with this form or online at:
http://www.haworthpress.com/store/product.asp?sku=5389

Diversity and Aging in the Social Environment

___ in softbound at $17.95 (ISBN: 0-7890-2676-7)
___ in hardbound at $29.95 (ISBN: 0-7890-2675-9)

COST OF BOOKS _____

POSTAGE & HANDLING _____
US: $4.00 for first book & $1.50
for each additional book
Outside US: $5.00 for first book
& $2.00 for each additional book.

SUBTOTAL _____

In Canada: add 7% GST. _____

STATE TAX _____
CA, IL, IN, MN, NJ, NY, OH & SD residents
please add appropriate local sales tax.

FINAL TOTAL _____
If paying in Canadian funds, convert
using the current exchange rate,
UNESCO coupons welcome.

❑ BILL ME LATER:
Bill-me option is good on US/Canada/
Mexico orders only; not good to jobbers,
wholesalers, or subscription agencies.

❑ Signature _____

❑ Payment Enclosed: $ _____

❑ PLEASE CHARGE TO MY CREDIT CARD:
❑ Visa ❑ MasterCard ❑ AmEx ❑ Discover
❑ Diner's Club ❑ Eurocard ❑ JCB

Account # _____

Exp Date _____

Signature _____
(Prices in US dollars and subject to change without notice.)

PLEASE PRINT ALL INFORMATION OR ATTACH YOUR BUSINESS CARD
Name
Address
City   State/Province   Zip/Postal Code
Country
Tel   Fax
E-Mail

May we use your e-mail address for confirmations and other types of information? ❑ Yes ❑ No We appreciate receiving
your e-mail address. Haworth would like to e-mail special discount offers to you, as a preferred customer.
We will never share, rent, or exchange your e-mail address. We regard such actions as an invasion of your privacy.

Order From Your **Local Bookstore** or Directly From
The Haworth Press, Inc. 10 Alice Street, Binghamton, New York 13904-1580 • USA
Call Our toll-free number (1-800-429-6784) / Outside US/Canada: (607) 722-5857
Fax: 1-800-895-0582 / Outside US/Canada: (607) 771-0012
E-mail your order to us: orders@haworthpress.com

For orders outside US and Canada, you may wish to order through your local
sales representative, distributor, or bookseller.
For information, see http://haworthpress.com/distributors

(Discounts are available for individual orders in US and Canada only, not booksellers/distributors.)

Please photocopy this form for your personal use.
www.HaworthPress.com   BOF05